Contents

Acknowledgements

This publication was written collectively by UFM network members during the period 2005-6.

Our heartfelt thanks go to everyone in UFM groups and beyond who has made time to share their personal experiences of working with UFM. Their contributions have been an invaluable guide to the authors in writing this book.

We would like to also thank:

Rosie Davies for her thoughtful comments

Patience Seebohm, Premila Trivedi and Frank Keating for their support and encouragement when the going was tough

Diana Rose for her continued support and her valuable advice

Lesley Warner for her help in looking at drafts

The Sainsbury Centre for Mental Health for funding UFM over the years and for publishing this guide and, in particular, we would like to thank Julie Hadman for seeing it through the production process.

This publication is dedicated to all those people who identify as service users or survivors of mental health services.

A Guide to User-Focused Monitoring

Setting up and running a project

Nutan Kotecha, Chandra Fowler, Anne-Laure Donskoy, Peter Johnson, Torsten Shaw, Karen Doherty

Other contributors:
Julia von Hausenchild, Krys Farrell, Graham Saxton, Shelley Welton, Derek Williams

ISBN13: 978 1 870480 71 0

Published by
The Sainsbury Centre for Mental Health
134-138 Borough High Street
London SE1 1LB
Tel: 020 7827 8300
Fax: 020 7403 9482
www.scmh.org.uk

The Sainsbury Centre for Mental Health (SCMH) is a charity that works to improve the quality of life for people with severe mental health problems. SCMH was founded in 1985 by the Gatsby Charitable Foundation, one of the Sainsbury Family Charitable Trusts, from which it receives core funding. SCMH is affiliated to the Institute of Psychiatry at King's College, London.

A charitable company limited by guarantee registered in England and Wales no. 4373019
Charity registration no. 1091156

Design: www.intertype.com
Printing: Nuffield Press, UK

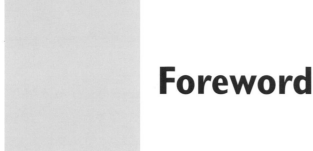

Foreword

Mental health services look very different according to one's position in relation to them: the perspective of those who provide them is poles apart from that of people who are on the receiving end of their ministrations, and differs again from the perspective of their relatives and friends. Historically the views of service providers have been the primary, and often the only, consideration. Service recipients were typically deemed incapable of expressing a cogent or meaningful perspective. 'Lack of insight' was deemed to be part and parcel of their illness, so their opinions were dismissed as nothing more than a reflection of their underlying pathology.

But over the last 30 years things have been changing. The demands of an increasingly vociferous and influential user/survivor movement in the 1980s have led to ever-greater attention being paid to the experience of using mental health services. The vision for the 'modernisation' of services presented in the *NHS Plan* (DH, 2000) and in the *National Service Framework for Mental Health* (DH, 1999), and reflected in all subsequent policy guidance, has at its core the requirement that services be tailored around the wishes, preferences and needs of those who use them, to create a patient-led NHS (DH, 2005a) that people have a positive experience of using.

Although we are clearly a long way from achieving this vision, obtaining the views of those who use the services is an increasingly important way of evaluating that quality. At a national level, the Healthcare Commission has conducted annual surveys of the views of those who use community services, and in 2007 it will also carry out an inpatient survey. At a local level, numerous attempts of varying quality have been made to provide individual teams and facilities with feedback about what they ought to do differently.

Service users have always been 'involved' in these surveys but traditionally only as respondents to the enquiries of clinicians and researchers. It remains the norm for clinicians and researchers to design questionnaires, interviews and inventories that reflect their own interests and concerns, which may or may not reflect the priorities of service users. Many service users remain reluctant to be open about their opinions for fear that this might have a negative impact on the support they receive, and all data obtained in the surveys is analysed and reported from within the parameters determined by the service provider.

The development of user-focused monitoring (UFM) at the Sainsbury Centre for Mental Health represents a radical departure from this tradition. The team responsible for this initiative was led by Dr Diana Rose, herself both a qualified researcher and a long-term user of both inpatient and community mental health services. It started from the premise that if the evaluation of services was genuinely to reflect the concerns and views of the people who use them rather than those of providers, then users should lead the process at every stage: from the questions asked, through the collection, analysis and interpretation of data to the final reporting of the results and development of recommendations for change.

UFM offers two types of information: the qualitative information necessary to inform providers about the types of changes that are needed, and the quantitative information necessary to evaluate the impact on the experience of using an individual service of any changes that have been made. Therefore, by repeating the process at regular intervals a team or service can progressively implement user-focused practice and service developments, and evaluate the impact of these on user experience in a continuing cycle of improvement.

We sincerely hope that this guide is widely used by service providers, commissioners, clinicians, researchers and service users to improve the quality of services. The people who use mental health services are the most important people in them (DH, 2000). It is only through this type of process that we can ever hope to achieve the vision of genuinely user-centred services tailored to the needs and preferences of those who use them.

Julie Repper,
Principal Research Fellow, Sheffield Hallam University

Rachel Perkins,
Director of Quality Assurance and User/Carer Experience,
South West London & St George's Mental Health NHS Trust

Introduction

“_Evaluation is exciting work that can really make you think about what you are doing and why._**”**

(Mckie et al., 2002)

About this guide

This book is essential reading for all those who wish to ensure that the service user's voice is heard in evaluations of mental health services. It provides a guide to setting up and running a user-focused monitoring (UFM) project where teams of service users are trained to interview other users about their experiences.

It has been written by people who have been involved in the development and delivery of UFM. They describe the practical challenges they have faced and how these were resolved. A list of essential criteria for UFM projects has been developed as a result of their experiences (see page 10) and this guide shows how these can be put into practice.

The guide is aimed at service users and mental health staff, including practitioners, managers and commissioners, who wish to set up a UFM project or find out more about the process. It will also be of interest to voluntary sector organisations that wish to support or develop a UFM project.

What is UFM?

UFM is a way of carrying out research in which the people who use mental health services evaluate the experiences of other mental health service users. It can be used both in the community and in hospital. It aims to put service users at the heart of the process and to improve the quality of mental health service delivery. It may also be a useful way of generating creative alternatives to the services that exist now.

The idea of service user involvement in mental health service development and practice is now firmly established. However, there are still serious questions as to its consistency and effectiveness (Trivedi, 2001; Trivedi _et al._, 2002; Oliver, 1992), and there are few examples of involvement moving beyond consultation to control. A greater understanding of the complexity of user involvement together with what needs to be put in place to support it properly (HASCAS, 2005) may now be emerging.

All UFM interviewees and interviewers are service users (many with severe mental health problems). Service users lead each stage of the UFM evaluation process (see Figure 1). UFM enables a wide range of service users whose voices are rarely sought to contribute their views, experiences and ideas to the evaluation process. This means reaching out to, among others, Black and minority ethnic (BME) people, those from refugee, gay and lesbian or homeless communities, individuals with physical or multiple disabilities and those who are economically and socially deprived.

> ❝ *We know from our experience that engaging patients and members of the public leads to research that is more relevant to people's needs and concerns, more reliable and more likely to be put into practice.* ❞

(DH, 2006a)

Powerful systems of exclusion particularly affect marginalised groups and explain why these tend to be present in the poorest (in terms of quality) parts of the mental health system. This creates ever-deepening exclusion and isolation and can lead to coercion and abuse within services (SCMH, 2002; Fernando, 2003; Williams & Keating, 2005).

People with mental health problems have also traditionally fared particularly badly in mainstream mental health research, which has been dominated by medical issues such as diagnosis and drug-based interventions. In this research, people who have mental health problems are 'subjects' who are researched and assessed in terms of their propensity to 'mental illness', with little regard to how they are affected by social and economic deprivation.

Service users and survivors have come up with a range of responses to being treated in this way (Pilgrim, 2005). UFM is one of these responses.

In traditional, professionally run evaluation interviews, service users are hesitant to be too open about their experiences. UFM has clearly shown (Rose, 2001) that if research is designed and conducted by service users it provides information that seldom emerges from more traditional research. Such information is essential if services are to become truly user-centred and driven by the needs, vision and creativity of those who most frequently use them.

> ❝ *My worst nightmare for UFM is that it is seen like a pretty butterfly that does nothing, a nice ornament. It's about people who have used mental health services, and often had a bad time of it, coming together to produce something that's useful, and that produces change.* ❞

UFM group member

Benefits of UFM

Over the last ten years, UFM has been developed at many sites in the UK. It has been shown to:

❖ provide an opportunity for people to lead and carry out an evaluation of a mental health service (drawing on their personal experience of services);

❖ enable the voices of marginalised service users to be heard and to influence service development;

❖ provide new perspectives and information to service providers;

❖ provide a crucial 'tool' for clinical governance;

❖ actively enable the development of equitable and constructive working partnerships between people who use services, service providers and commissioners and wider communities within a locality.

> ❝ *My self-confidence and self-esteem, absolutely at nil when I first became involved with UFM, have had a tremendous boost and I have found that I have used organising skills I didn't know I had. I have made great friends within the team and have had many laughs. I appreciate the help and support everyone offers, not just to me, but also to each other. It has also been good to see other members of the team using their old and new skills.* ❞

UFM group member

Where UFM is carried out in accordance with the principles set out in this guide, it also brings direct benefits to service users involved in UFM groups, by:

❖ providing an opportunity to do something that values personal experiences;

❖ reducing isolation and providing an opportunity to make new friends;

❖ participating in an activity that is not about being helped but helping others;

❖ earning money;

❖ developing skills and confidence.

How it all began

The idea of UFM was developed at the Sainsbury Centre for Mental Health (SCMH) in 1996 and, originally, UFM projects were co-ordinated directly by members of the UFM team based there. Findings from these early reports are presented in an earlier publication, *Users' Voices* (Rose, 2001).

From 2002, as new UFM projects were set up, co-ordinators were recruited locally, with 'arm's length' support available from the UFM co-ordinator at SCMH. Soon after, a national UFM Network was set up specifically to support local UFM projects and to enable UFM co-ordinators and group members to network and share experiences and progressively refine the process of UFM. During this time, both the co-ordinator at SCMH and the UFM Network received many requests for information and advice about UFM, not only from individual service users and service users' groups but also from NHS managers, clinicians and commissioners of services. It also became apparent that some projects identifying themselves as UFM projects were being undertaken in less than desirable ways and not in accordance with the principles that had been developed and then set out in *Users' Voices*. In response to this it was decided to produce an accessible and comprehensive guide setting out the practice, achievements and challenges of UFM.

The UFM approach is part of a much broader development, in which people who identify themselves as survivors and/or service users carry out research within mental health services, covering issues that range much wider than services themselves, such as employment, self-definitions of distress, coping strategies and alternatives to medical treatment.

We want to acknowledge the fact that many of the ideas developed for UFM and set out in this guide have their roots in the ground-breaking research emerging from the emancipation and disability movements of the 1960s and 1970s (Turner & Beresford, 2005). This work provided the foundation for the development of service user research. It is important to remember that UFM is only one approach to service user-led research; it does not claim to be the only or the right way.

At the same time, whatever the nature of service provision in years to come, the need for services to be evaluated from the standpoint of people who use them has never been greater. This is a political issue. There remains a huge chasm between the political imperatives of managing risk and the imperatives of creating services that are enabling and provide real support, sanctuary and safety. Establishing and sustaining UFM projects has involved great struggle which will continue just as struggles continue in user involvement generally and in user-led research.

Essential criteria for UFM projects

A list of essential criteria for UFM projects has been developed by the UFM Network, based on their experiences in setting up and running projects. These are derived from a list first published in *Doing it for Real* (UFM Network, 2003).

1. Projects should be led and controlled by service users. This means, for example, that:

   ❖ the research topic is chosen on the basis of the concerns of local service users;

   ❖ the questions are created by service users with reference to and input from a range of people using the services under evaluation (e.g. people outside the UFM group itself);

   ❖ service users form at least one-half (plus one person) of any management structure, e.g. steering group;

   ❖ service users are actively encouraged and supported to take part at all stages of the project.

   In circumstances where it has not been immediately possible to recruit a co-ordinator with personal experience of using services or mental health difficulties, UFM co-ordinators must have a demonstrable understanding of and commitment to service user research and involvement, and a commitment to working towards UFM becoming a fully service user-controlled project.

2. There should be a clear focus on the development and improvement of those services that are most frequently used by service users, particularly those from marginalised groups.

3. There should be an active commitment to secure the participation (as UFM group members/ researchers and wider contributors) of (a large proportion of) service users who have used the services under evaluation, including those people whose voices are rarely heard.

   The project should provide opportunities for individual service users to be involved in a variety of ways and at different levels in the research process, for instance, question development, data input, analysis, writing the report and recommendations for change, dissemination and implementation process. All service users (including interviewees) should be appropriately paid for their input and have their reasonable expenses reimbursed.

   Service providers and others involved in the project (e.g. steering or advisory group members) should be active in promoting UFM within services and be proactive in supporting it to achieve and maintain its principles, particularly in relation to following through recommendations to achieve positive change.

4. There should be an aim to disseminate findings as widely as possible, including ensuring that all interviewees receive feedback on the findings of the evaluation and are invited to give their views on the process and outcomes. Allies within mental health services and funders should provide support for this.

5. There should be a commitment to addressing equalities issues, e.g. by ensuring that the views and opinions of those people whose voices are rarely heard are included, as members of the UFM group and as participants (i.e. those being interviewed). These may include:

   ❖ people who have been threatened with or have experienced compulsory treatment;

   ❖ people who are perceived as 'difficult to manage', too ill or too 'dangerous';

   ❖ people with disabilities, including those with multiple or invisible disabilities;

❖ Black and minority ethnic (BME) and Irish communities;

❖ people who have complained about or who have disengaged from mental health services;

as well as many other excluded groups (UFM Network, 2003).

It is important to remember that there is a distinction between those people who identify as service users who are involved in creating and shaping the UFM process (e.g. as members of the group and interviewers) and those who are participants in the evaluation itself (i.e. those who are interviewed). Both groups will include people who have had significant mental health problems.

UFM works as an enabling group process, designed to ensure that UFM principles (including those of equality and open access for all) are upheld and that the focus of the project is maintained. The co-ordinator is accountable to the UFM group and is fundamentally a facilitator, although responsible, together with any steering or advisory group, for ensuring that UFM principles are adhered to. There should be regular opportunities for new people to join the group.

6. There should be independence, with the UFM group and co-ordinator having control over key decision-making areas such as timescales for projects and budgets, with the freedom to write and publish their findings without interference. True independence cannot be achieved without secure and adequate funding, e.g. to employ the UFM co-ordinator, to pay service user project workers and other costs, and to allow sufficient time to take the project to completion.

7. The UFM group should develop and follow good standards of research methodology (see Chapter 8).

8. The co-ordinator and project group should receive supervision and support, with access to appropriate expertise, throughout the UFM project. This should be flexible to allow for differing levels of experience, strengths and skills.

9. Accessible, flexible and comprehensive training should be available for the whole project team, including the co-ordinator, catering for the different needs of the service users involved.

10. There should be a commitment to implementing the recommendations from commissioners and service providers. This should be demonstrated by planning the process for implementation as early as possible and making resources available for it, including for the involvement of service users.

Figure 1: Overview of the process of a UFM project

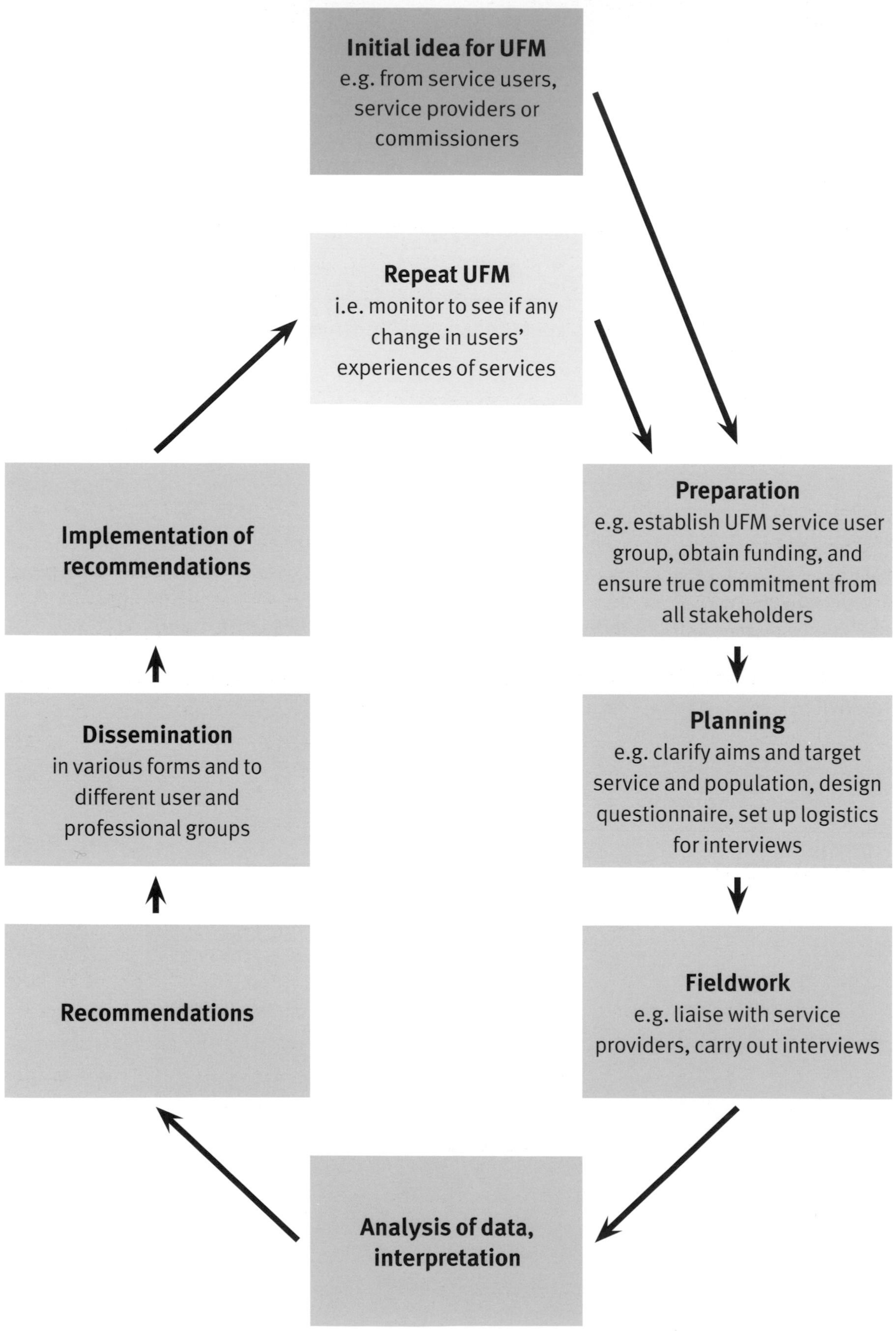

Initial idea for UFM
e.g. from service users, service providers or commissioners

Repeat UFM
i.e. monitor to see if any change in users' experiences of services

Implementation of recommendations

Preparation
e.g. establish UFM service user group, obtain funding, and ensure true commitment from all stakeholders

Dissemination
in various forms and to different user and professional groups

Planning
e.g. clarify aims and target service and population, design questionnaire, set up logistics for interviews

Recommendations

Fieldwork
e.g. liaise with service providers, carry out interviews

Analysis of data, interpretation

CHAPTER 1

Diversity, inequalities and power imbalances

Introduction

People using mental health services come from many different backgrounds. This can have a big effect on how they experience mental health care. People from African and Caribbean communities, for example, are much more likely than others to come into contact with the service through the police and under the Mental Health Act. When using services they are over-represented in hospital and in secure services (SCMH, 2006).

These issues must be considered carefully at the outset of any UFM project. The project needs to work positively to reflect the diversity of the population using the service and to value the experiences of everyone involved.

In a social context, the term '*diversity*' refers to all the ways in which people within a population are different from one another, e.g. in terms of age, 'race', ethnicity, class, sex, physical abilities/qualities, sexual orientation, religion, gender expression, educational background, income, etc. In UFM projects there is also diversity, for example, in terms of personal experience of mental health problems and mental health services, interpretations of mental health problems, diagnosis and treatment.

The views and concerns of certain groups still tend to be under-represented in research. These groups also tend to be under-represented in most user organisations and 'user involvement' exercises. Recommendations have been made for the establishment of separate Black user groups to encourage BME users to become more involved in mental health service development (Wallcraft *et al.*, 2003).

Power imbalances

UFM, with its strong service user focus, seeks to redress some of the imbalances in power which have traditionally existed between mental health service users and providers and to enable service users to take control over the way in which the services they receive are developed. In addition in UFM, there will not only be diversity and power differentials between users and mental health professionals, but also between those within each group. All aspects of UFM must therefore be mindful of issues of diversity and equality. However, there may be certain areas where this will be of particular importance, for example in:

❖ the way the specific subject area of UFM is chosen;

❖ how the project is supervised, steered or advised and by whom;

❖ the way the group is led and works together;

❖ what support and adaptations are available to facilitate the involvement of marginalised groups;

❖ how decisions are made;

❖ what type of training is given and who delivers it;

❖ who has access to what information.

So, placing diversity and equality at the forefront of any UFM project provides a very useful and constructive way of identifying and working to address the very considerable power differentials that exist in mental health services.

Experience has shown that such opportunities may be difficult to open up. However, this is not an area that should be seen as an 'optional extra' and no progress will be made if it is avoided or not even on the agenda.

Box 1 describes the experiences of a Black service user facilitating a 'Letting Through Light' (LTL) project which has conducted two audits to involve BME communities in planning and developing mental health services (Ferns, 2003).

Box 1: Experiences of a Black service user facilitator

I worked on the first Letting Through Light (LTL) project (Ferns & Trivedi, 2002) which, although not UFM, was loosely built on and adapted from a UFM-type process.

Some of the particular challenges that we faced and worked with included the following:

Consideration of precisely what we meant by 'BME' communities

This collective term covers a very wide range of communities in England, with very diverse experiences of life, mental distress and the mental health system. We soon realised that if our 'BME' project was to be meaningful we would have to define precisely which communities (or groups of communities) we were working with.

In our first audit project in Birmingham we worked specifically with African, Caribbean and South Asian service users. The second audit included Irish service users, since the local user organisation we were working through had clear concerns about how this community experienced mental health services.

Working with 'BME' service users from very diverse communities

We were working with communities who had quite different issues with the mental health system, did not normally work together and (in some cases) had quite stereotyped views about one another. We allowed lots of time for people to begin to get to know one another in a safe setting and identify commonalities that would enable them to work together while still recognising and respecting their differences. It was both challenging and very exciting to see service users from very different communities getting to know each other, challenging their own stereotypes and identifying common experiences that would enable them to build new and successful working relationships. Time and resources were critical in enabling this to happen.

Working with difficult feelings based on experience of services

Raising the possibility of BME service users bringing about improvements in mental health services was often understandably met with derision and cynicism, with Black users angrily asking how they could possibly believe they could bring about change in services when they could never get staff to listen to their concerns about their treatment.

Box 1: Experiences of a Black service user facilitator *(continued)*

We learned that those Black service users whose basic needs (e.g. for support with housing, benefits and medication) had been denied were left in a position where they might not have the resources, energy or inclination to be involved in LTL. Our response was to validate those experiences by enabling those people who felt angry and let down to express their feelings and tell their story in whatever way they wanted. The importance of this became clearer as we saw a very gradual shift, with people beginning to channel these experiences through the audit.

Recognising that being a Black service user yourself is not always enough

When I got involved in the first LTL project, I expected that the BME service users we worked with would openly accept us and trust that we had a commitment to bringing about change in mental health services. I was completely unprepared for the criticisms directed at us, which at some points included accusations that we had been sucked in and become part of the mental health system.

My colleagues and I realised that we had to take on board these negative feelings towards us and work through them. Recognising where these strong antagonistic feelings were coming from, acknowledging people's right to have such feelings, trying not to be defensive, taking a less structured stance, being very open about our own experiences and being prepared to step out of our 'leading the project' role certainly helped. Trust, friendship and humour slowly built up among the group during some fiery and exhausting days.

Key lessons

There are a number of ways in which UFM projects can work positively with diversity. Some of the key lessons learned from previous projects are listed here.

Create space for discussion

Find time and ways to create space for all those involved in the project to have general and non-threatening conversations about their attitude to diversity and inequalities. These conversations should also look at ways of tackling any issues that arise.

This process is never easy and will need to be skilfully facilitated to ensure that people stay with the process and don't end up being excluded or excluding themselves. Here it may be important for the UFM co-ordinator to take a strong and confident leadership role and to bring in additional support as necessary. Service users in the group may be very committed to asserting the rights of service users in a mental health context. However, they may not always be so aware of or passionate about asserting the rights of marginalised groups or the rights of various groups of other service users – for example, they may have prejudices about self-harm.

Provide opportunities to learn

There are many ways in which people can gain knowledge about issues of diversity and equality. It can be useful to have accessible and relevant literature and resources such as books, poetry and videos/DVDs that can be lent to people or shown to the group. These could be resources produced within the mental health field, and in particular those by users/survivors, which often cover many aspects of social inequality and related power dynamics within mental health services, in accessible ways. Other relevant resources on diversity and equality may include those from feminist, gay, anti-racist and physical disability arenas.

Plan time to reflect

Allowing time to reflect on what has been happening within a project at certain times can help people to learn about issues of diversity and equalities. Moreover, taking time to find out what is happening enables appropriate action to be taken. For example, if several people from a specific 'sub-group', e.g. younger people, are dropping out of a steering group or project team, perhaps there is a problem that needs to be faced: maybe they are feeling excluded or lack confidence. Considering such issues sensitively and openly as they arise will do much to prevent people feeling alienated or thinking that the group is not accessible to them.

Acknowledge power differences

In UFM as in any other (service user) group, power differentials can exist even within the group and between the co-ordinator and the group. This needs to be acknowledged (Mental Health Foundation, 2003).

Value people's different skills and interests

UFM is not only about the mechanics of the research process. It is important to value all roles within the group and match skills and interest to opportunities. Value is often reflected in terms of payment and status, so if you are paying only those people who are doing interviews, be aware of the message this can give.

All service users should have equal access to the opportunities that UFM offers. It can be very easy to give certain types of work to people who already have skills, which may mean that others do not get the opportunity to learn them.

Offer choices – don't make assumptions

All interviewees need to be offered an interview with someone of the same sex (and if possible and so desired, with other shared grounds, e.g. sexuality or ethnic origin). Never assume, however, that this is what people want. Give people a choice wherever possible. Alison Faulkner, writing in *The Ethics of Survivor Research*, gives an example of a scenario of South Asian interviewees preferring to be interviewed by someone from a non-Asian background: "Boundaries of knowledge and confidentiality can be more complex in smaller communities where knowledge might be shared" (Faulkner, 2004).

> **"***Diversity is then not just about tolerating difference, but about developing a set of conscious and active practices which recognise and welcome difference and the consequences (and benefits!) it may have on people's lives. Diversity is also not just about those we perceive as different, but is about everybody working together to create inclusive, respectful and equitable communities. This is particularly important within mental health services, where the massive and institutionalised power imbalances between service providers and service users often leave service users feeling disempowered, defeated and/or angry.***"**

Black service user trainer

CHAPTER 2

Getting started

This chapter looks at the issues that need to be considered and addressed when trying to get a UFM project off the ground. As UFM projects begin in different ways, there is no step-by-step guide, but there are some common areas.

Preparation

Everything will take a long time at first. Building up good contacts is essential. Don't give up and be prepared for peaks and troughs.

Service user

Good preparation pays dividends later in a UFM project. Key points to consider when starting a project include:

- making contact with other UFM projects to get support and information;
- how to generate a broad base of enthusiasm, support and commitment for UFM;
- how to involve people;
- how to manage the project;
- how to address issues of diversity, inequalities and power imbalances;
- what supports or expertise are needed;
- how to obtain and manage funding;
- how to maintain independence and user control of the project;
- how to decide the subject area of the evaluation;
- how progress will be reviewed;
- setting up supports for group members.

Finding your allies

The support of sympathetic and interested mental health workers is important in order to promote a broader understanding and acceptance of UFM among other professionals. With their assistance it will be much easier to gain the support of senior managers and commissioners; you may already have identified service providers or commissioners who are sympathetic to the idea of UFM, which will make the task much easier.

"UFM could be in danger of getting used as a tick box exercise. My advice is to look for those people who believe it is important to make it happen, who will be able to assist in securing resources and dealing with problems, but will not want to exert control of it as a result. "

UFM co-ordinator

Think about those professionals who have a good 'track record' of supporting true 'service user' involvement, and those who are unhappy with the way services currently work. It may also be useful to develop a campaign to gain publicity and support.

"The UFM project has become an integral part of responsive commissioning of mental health services. My role has been to champion UFM, promoting it throughout our PCT and partner agencies and chairing meetings of the steering group where action plans responding to the findings are developed and monitored. As well as the many changes to policy and practice that UFM has brought about at our local mental health trust, the project has had an important impact here at the PCT. The UFM project has served as a guide to other user involvement initiatives and policies such as the PCT's service user payments policy. "

Director of service development in a primary care trust (PCT)

Box 2: Clinical lead nurse on a UFM evaluation of residential services

We wanted to find ways of developing devolved decision-making, staff and user empowerment and partnership working in our unit which consists of three residential homes within an NHS trust. Funding was provided by the trust's audit department and a UFM worker was seconded for one day a week.

At the beginning of this process, it was acknowledged that staff were committed to the idea of service user involvement and had supported the development of residents' meetings, involvement of service users in staff recruitment and surveys of users' views of services. While still valuable, the leadership team considered some of these processes to be rather tokenistic. If we were honest, we recognised that the agendas for change were generally staff-driven and that when we sought the views of service users only a few people (usually the same few) took part.

We realised that if we really wanted to know what residents thought of the services they received, then we needed to find a way of involving more residents in the process as well as assuring their anonymity.

The UFM project which evaluated us has so far exceeded our expectations in terms of providing objective and meaningful feedback on services provided. It has become an invaluable resource in accessing and representing the views of people who use the residential services. Members of the team now sit on the Practice Development Unit Council to ensure that recommendations from the evaluation findings are put into practice and followed through.

The UFM project has continued to grow and strengthen in its passion to influence service development. It has continued to provide both support for positive developments and constructive challenge where needed. We would like to see the UFM project expanding into education and research as well as continuing to take part in evaluation of services and ensuring that recommendations for change are followed through.

The project has provided employment opportunities for people who use mental health services. The team members have provided hope and inspiration to other service users they have interviewed.

Publicity and recruitment

Making local service users, providers and commissioners and staff aware of what UFM is, what is involved and what it can achieve can have a number of positive results. It may open up access to the right contacts within the services being evaluated, and help adequate funding to be agreed at an early stage. Local service users may be more willing to become involved when they know that UFM can be effective in driving change. It is important to:

❖ be explicit about how UFM could be used to improve local mental health services, maybe raising some issues that are known to be of local concern and how UFM could be used to address these. Demonstrating the existence of this commitment is likely to be critical, particularly if there is distrust about any change that has emerged from other schemes in the past;

❖ bring in examples of where UFM has been used in other places to bring about improvements in services and/or invite in others to talk briefly about their experiences of being involved in UFM;

❖ describe how UFM is led by local service users and provides them with opportunities to become involved in ways that are of personal benefit to them;

❖ provide some simple handouts for people to take away and read in their own time.

Box 3: UFM co-ordinator on starting a project

It is important to consider how the benefits of UFM can be conveyed to local service users, providers and commissioners. This may be done by bringing people together at an informal 'gathering' or by going to a place where people who use services gather, whether it's a day centre, a ward or a social group.

As a newly appointed UFM co-ordinator, one of my first tasks was to find out whether there was an active mental health service user community. Had anyone heard of UFM before? What user involvement initiatives had been undertaken in the past?

I found out there was lots of potential. Many people within services knew all about UFM. There were some service user groups linked to the voluntary organisations but no actual involvement in planning mental health services had been sustained. Those who had been involved in previous initiatives had become frustrated and disillusioned.

My supervisor, an experienced UFM co-ordinator, suggested that I start with building some awareness. I decided to arrange an event about 'Mental health and wellbeing' with music, food, displays and complementary therapies. This included a 'chat room' where people could relax and find out about UFM. We also provided a 'Sound-off tree' on the wall where people could use coloured 'stickies' to say what they thought about local services.

We raised the profile of UFM and got a number of people to join the UFM group. By providing an environment where people with mental health problems felt relaxed and weren't being asked to 'do anything' or 'represent anyone', we were able to get more people to attend than if it had been a service user involvement event. We also got some interesting feedback on local mental health services and promoted the importance of mental health and wellbeing to a wide audience.

Opportunities should also be provided for interested practitioners, managers and/or commissioners to learn about UFM, its philosophy and potential, either with service users or on their own, depending on what will work best in the local context. Discussing local issues and hearing users' experiences and views on services may be challenging for service providers and commissioners, but also enlightening, and it is an essential part of the UFM process. Reaching shared agreements later in the process about how a UFM project should be run will be much easier if early frank communication has occurred and the principles and ethos of UFM have been fully subscribed to.

Focus on local service users' agendas

When you have a group of service users who are interested in taking the project forward it will be essential to have an open and honest discussion so that people can talk about their experiences of local services and highlight their concerns.

People often have had few chances to discuss what has happened to them in a sympathetic setting, and there is bound to be a lot of anger and pain. People need these opportunities so that they can start to move away from being fixed on their own experience to thinking more broadly about services and their impact. Good facilitation skills, sensitivity and time will be essential for these discussions, which can often be challenging but also energising and unifying for service users.

Although other service users may not become directly involved at this stage, it is crucial to ensure that they are kept informed and updated about any UFM project that is developed, so that a wide base of support is established and a sense of ownership generated within the local service user community. In addition, it may well be necessary at various stages of the project to call upon the interest, co-operation and involvement of local service users not directly involved in the UFM project, and this will be much easier if they are already informed and involved to some degree. Finally, regular updates and open communication may also help prevent some of the tensions and conflict that can arise when (as has sometimes happened) UFM is perceived to be affecting the funding and support of other service user groups or projects in the area.

Applying for and obtaining funding

Securing adequate funding to carry out the UFM project and see it through to its conclusion is essential, and the source, amount and duration of funding will influence what you can realistically do within the UFM project. It is therefore sensible to secure funding before planning the UFM project further. This guide, together with *Users' Voices* (Rose, 2001), will provide enough background information to produce a funding application to present to potential funding bodies.

Most UFM projects are now funded by local primary care trusts (PCTs), and where mental health services are provided across several PCTs, more than one PCT may be involved. Some UFM projects have been funded directly by NHS mental health trusts or local authorities, and a few by voluntary sector organisations. In all cases, funders have varied in how much freedom they have given the UFM project to decide on its focus and how the funding is spent.

Box 4: The challenge of maintaining funding

A service user research forum hosted by a local mental health trust with representatives from various user groups campaigned for a user-led UFM project. Two local PCTs agreed to fund this project and allowed voluntary sector organisations to bid for the contract. A local voluntary sector organisation, composed mainly of service users, was awarded one year's funding after an arduous selection process. The success of the first project led to the PCT agreeing a service-level agreement for future years.

Ensuring actual security was very difficult, however, as no definite duration of funding had been agreed and small under-spends on the budget made it difficult to argue for continuation of funding at the same level. A contract was negotiated that required the PCT to give at least six months' notice if it intended to stop the funding. The project had strong service user control and was supported by a host organisation with a strong user-led ethos. The host organisation was a relatively stable voluntary sector organisation with several other projects and an infrastructure to support these projects. There were also a number of notable allies in the PCTs, local mental health trust and elsewhere who gave their support.

Adequate and secure funding is an essential prerequisite for any UFM project. Although projects may vary, funding is required to cover the following:

❖ employment of a UFM project co-ordinator for at least four days a week (salary, employer costs, pension) plus expenses (e.g. travel costs);

❖ set-up costs (e.g. computer and office equipment);

❖ payment to host organisation (e.g. rent, stationery, heating, lighting, administrative resources, managerial support, telephone, photocopier, postage);

❖ workers' costs (payments plus expenses);

❖ training for co-ordinator and workers;

❖ support and supervision of co-ordinator and workers;

❖ recruitment of participants and payment for their time and travel;

❖ printing and dissemination of report;

❖ involvement in implementation process.

66 I think it is really important to think about funding strategies and independence. Getting grants for pieces of work may provide a more stable foundation but does make you much more under the control of grant issuers and makes you vulnerable if the funding stops or is cut. The advantage of charging for work that people approach you to do is greater flexibility about what you do and what you don't; it also helps clarify exactly what work you are doing. 99

UFM co-ordinator

UFM projects currently operate with different amounts of funding. The UFM Network believes that funding of £55,000 a year (2006 figures) is needed for an adequately funded UFM project to develop and maintain a firm foundation and a good standard of work.

UFM is intended to be a cyclical process and this clearly has implications for the duration of funding, which ideally should be ongoing and indefinite.

In pilot UFM projects, 12 months tended to be a popular duration, but this puts great pressure on the process and severely limits the ability of projects to support the implementation of their findings.

Box 5: UFM member on sustainability and funding

The members of our UFM group were recruited by the local user involvement organisation. All of us had been 'survivors' from a prior (and much derided) audit. After two UFM projects, the parent organisation of our research group was dissolved. But we were not too apprehensive about the idea of independence and some of us saw it as a positive development.

Our research group survived and continued to work, completing a third piece of work. Members believed this was possibly due to our semi-autonomy and principles of democracy, based on 100% consensus and equality.

However, between projects we really struggled to maintain ourselves as a group of volunteers. At this point, we felt the absence of a co-ordinator: there was no funding between projects and no one to support the group or negotiate new research. The loss of the parent organisation also meant that we did not have the opportunity to take part in other work or training.

Having tried to continue our work as a research group with some *ad hoc* support, we have realised this is not sustainable in the long term. We have learned that without proper levels of support and funding, maintaining a user-led group that produces a high standard of work is extremely difficult.

A cautionary note is needed here: where funding is in principle agreed over a three-year cycle, it is essential that this is reflected in a 'contract'. As in the example in Box 4, some projects have found that their funding had to be re-negotiated after a period of time because it had only been confirmed for the first year. Any contract should ensure that the funding body will give notice if it intends to cease funding, and that it will state how long the notice will be. We would suggest six months is reasonable and would allow the group to plan for the future.

The importance of allowing enough time

Perhaps the most important resource after funding for a UFM project is time, in terms not only of users' time but also that of service providers or commissioners.

Often, in user-led projects, the amount of time required to carry out the project is seriously under-estimated and can lead to serious frustration and burn-out. Proper consideration must be given to the time implications for any UFM project, e.g. time to ensure that users and professionals understand and are committed to the project, time for the researchers to be trained and to practise their new skills, time to carry out the interviews without feeling pressurised and rushed, time to debrief following interviews, time to consider and interpret the findings and, finally, time to make recommendations and disseminate the results.

Establishing a UFM steering or advisory group

Some UFM projects have steering groups or advisory groups. There are definite advantages to having a group that provides advice and support to a project.

Advisory groups have the advantage over steering groups of allowing overall control to lie with the service users within the UFM group while still being there as a support when needed.

Steering groups have an overall collective responsibility for ensuring that a project meets its objectives, and the decisions of a steering group are binding on the project. In theory, steering group members will take a more active role, owing to this greater responsibility for the project, but in practice this is by no means always the case. Members of an advisory group may also be willing to take a proactive role outside of the meetings, but this will need to be clarified in their terms of reference.

It is advisable when selecting members of an advisory or steering group to look for a good mix of effective people who can provide a range of inputs and perspectives. UFM group members and non-UFM service users should be present, as well as voluntary sector staff. Appendix 1 gives further guidance on setting up advisory/steering groups.

Deciding where to base the UFM project

UFM projects have been established in very different ways. Some projects have been located within a service user/survivor organisation or other local voluntary sector organisation such as an advocacy service; others have been located within a PCT or a mental health trust, or linked to a university. *Doing it for Real* (UFM Network, 2003) emphasised the importance of independence for UFM projects. It is likely to be easier to guarantee this in a service user/survivor organisation and in some voluntary sector organisations.

The independence of the project can be more difficult to guarantee if it is located within a mental health trust. This does not mean that mental health trusts should not fund projects. But it does mean that much thought needs to go into safeguarding independence. This could include providing funding through an independent organisation. One way in which this has been done is for a mental health trust to invite several interested organisations to prepare a written proposal about how they would support and run a UFM project and what they would charge for doing so. This process of applying for a contract to run any project or service is called tendering. Once the proposals are received the trust follows a selection process to choose the most suitable candidate.

If the independent organisation chosen is user-led or the majority of the leadership is in the hands of service users then this is also likely to encourage a culture in which the project group feels able to withstand the pressures that can occur when service users' agendas and priorities conflict with those of service providers or academics.

Major difficulties can arise for service user co-ordinators carrying out UFM in settings where they have themselves received treatment.

> *There have been many challenges for me in this UFM project. Some of these have been about the way the project was set up. Working with the same mental health trust and hospital where I spent most of my time as an inpatient has been difficult. From time to time, I have flashbacks of experiences from my stays there. I work in an office with a nurse who has nursed me in the past.*

*I go to the canteen and many of the people there have seen me in a patient role. Our office is even considering moving to the building where the old wards are. I could end up with an office which is in the same room where I was an inpatient!*99

UFM co-ordinator

CHAPTER 3

The UFM co-ordinator

This chapter looks at the role of the UFM co-ordinator and explains why a full-time post is needed. It identifies the key qualities required for a co-ordinator and examines the issues to be considered when recruiting.

66*UFM is hard work but doing it has been surprisingly a lot of fun too.*99

UFM co-ordinator

The co-ordinator is one of the most important assets for any UFM project and is usually recruited before the group is formed. This is because in the past there has been a tendency for funders/service providers to decide the initial area of research and to begin the project by recruiting the co-ordinator themselves.

It is now good practice in many mental health trusts to involve service users in the recruitment process. It is also advisable for co-ordinators coming into post to have the opportunity to consult with local service users about their priorities for evaluation. If the general focus has been decided, then they should ensure that the reasons for this are transparent.

However, there have been examples of a group of service users leading the recruitment of their co-ordinator. This has usually been in projects where service user groups have lobbied successfully for a project to begin.

66*Our research group was based within a broader service user involvement project and lost our co-ordinator when the project lost funding. We then set up as an independent research group and drew up our own recruitment criteria, interviewing the co-ordinator ourselves.*99

UFM group member

Role of co-ordinator

UFM is a service user-led initiative and the role of the co-ordinator must be clear. Co-ordinators should be responsible and accountable to the research group, viewing themselves essentially as facilitators.

Most past and current co-ordinators have been service users, or have experienced significant mental distress but have not had contact with mental health services. Ideally, recruitment should be aimed at people who have experienced mental health problems. However, there are some co-ordinators who have not had this experience, but have nevertheless successfully managed UFM projects. The key seems to be to ensure that co-ordinators have a demonstrable understanding of and commitment to service user-led projects. This understanding and commitment needs to be rigorously tested at the application and interview stages of the recruitment process.

The task of a UFM co-ordinator is a varied one which requires a range of distinct skills. Current co-ordinators feel that the most important skills are:

❖ the ability to support and facilitate a group of service user researchers;

❖ the ability to 'think on your feet', responding appropriately to problems as they arise;

❖ the confidence to say no if necessary when faced with demands from service users and staff to engage in wider user involvement;

❖ the ability to lead where necessary on equality and diversity issues and maintain the focus of the project.

Co-ordinators need a good understanding of how research is carried out as well as an understanding and awareness of the dynamics and complexity of implementing change within services. However, a vast amount of experience in these areas is not essential because good training, supervision and support can help the development of such skills, as well as refreshing a co-ordinator's understanding and ability to apply research methods and address equalities issues.

66 *It's been really good to see other service users from the group go on to run the project or on to other paid research posts.* 99

Former UFM co-ordinator

Recommended core skills/experience for the co-ordinator include:

❖ experience of service use and/or experience of working with service users in an equal, supportive and facilitative way;

❖ a strong awareness and appreciation of stigma and discrimination as experienced in mental health contexts (as well as by other communities) and a demonstrable commitment to equalities issues, with an appreciation of social and economic issues;

❖ understanding of and experience of research processes;

❖ ability to facilitate a group and work with group dynamics.

The co-ordinator may need some training before they begin work with the group as, indeed, may their manager.

Support and supervision

66 *Isolation perhaps has been the greatest obstacle for me so far, feeling isolated from other projects and workers. If you are a lone worker it's essential to find your support networks.* 99

New UFM co-ordinator

As well as support for the research process it is essential that co-ordinators have access to regular emotional support in the form of (at least) monthly external supervision. Both mental health services and the voluntary sector can be stressful places to work. UFM co-ordinators often find themselves at the interface of both these sectors. They can also find themselves isolated and caught between staff and service users. Creating an environment that is open and inviting, and dealing with any problems that may arise between service users, can be difficult.

66 *I am daunted and excited at the size of the task ahead: building a new team, getting organised, choosing the next subject for research, working on the implementation process of the last project and so on, but also looking after myself and my mental health, learning not to overwork (...too late already for that one!). It is a real challenge. Nonetheless that journey shows that a service user like me with no previous extensive research experience, but bringing a lot of enthusiasm and passion*

for user-led research, can look forward and defeat the usual low expectations that some have about long-term service users. UFM can be a pretty chaotic world but that is the attraction too!❯❯

UFM co-ordinator

A suitable external supervisor is likely to have extensive experience and knowledge of the voluntary or mental health service sectors, counselling skills, and a good understanding of how research and evaluation work. They also need to be independent of any organisations or groups that the co-ordinator will be engaging with. Previous UFM co-ordinators can be effective supervisors.

Box 6: The experiences of a UFM co-ordinator

The role of UFM co-ordinator initially focused on administrative work such as processing expenses, writing letters and arranging meetings. The project was managed by an external co-ordinator who provided the research experience, and an internal facilitator who had a full-time role within the mental health trust.

I wanted service users to own the project. We do have the skills already and the capability to pick up new skills. I gradually expanded my influence and role.

As I took on more elements of the management role, I had to work more hours (15 then 25 then 30) and develop the project's profile within the trust and outside. I now have someone who does my administrative work for ten hours per week. This in turn has brought new challenges such as supervision and work allocation.

We are currently funded for two projects per year but recently commissioners have approached us to carry out surveys in other areas of mental health care.

CHAPTER 4

The research group

Recruitment of the research group is a crucial stage in the UFM project, as the people in the group will be the ones carrying out most of the work. The aim is to recruit a group of between 10 and 14 people.

There are various ways of going about the process. It is important to consider equalities issues carefully but, at the same time, to be realistic in your aims. How you start off your recruitment will affect who is likely to get involved. Bear in mind that you are aiming to recruit a group who have some experience of the subject area of the project (if that has been decided).

It is important to make a special effort at an early stage to recruit from relevant groups such as service users from Black and minority ethnic (BME) communities and people who are less confident about coming forward and therefore less likely to join. The barriers to joining are likely to be higher once a group has formed.

If the project is applicable to a particular group, owing to the proposed subject of the evaluation, start recruiting those people first.

Overcoming barriers to participation

There are a number of things that can form a barrier:

Barriers of education

Research has tended to be seen as an academic activity that requires a high level of education. This is certainly not true for UFM which, though it requires some skills, emphasises the expertise that is gained by personal experience. Do not assume, however, that none of the service users showing an interest in UFM has a high level of education or skills. UFM projects should provide a variety of ways for people to get involved, including opportunities for people who have no research skills. It should even be possible to arrange for people with poor literacy skills to be involved in some way. Therefore invitations to participate should not only be in written format.

Barriers of bureaucracy

The way in which benefit regulations work at present has a negative impact on user involvement and individuals' willingness to become more active and therefore visible to the system. Members of the research group may have to carry out procedures in which they have to sign contracts, provide personal information and undergo a Criminal Records Bureau (CRB) check. Many service users have well-founded reasons to distrust organisational systems. Information, time, reassurance and support will be necessary.

Barriers of past and present circumstances

Particular groups of service users who have had difficult and painful experiences of mental health care may not feel enthusiastic or safe working on a project that deals directly with mental health services. Some groups of service users, in particular from BME communities, may be more reluctant than others to take part in such projects, because of their more frequent experiences of inappropriate treatment and coercion within services. In addition, if people are struggling in poverty and with problems concerning housing, etc. they may not be in a position to have a real choice about participating.

Trivedi and Keating state: "based on our experience of working with people from BME communities, it's hardly surprising that service users from BME communities do not become 'involved', when services repeatedly fail to meet even their most basic needs" (Trivedi & Keating, 2006).

Barriers of disillusionment and distrust

Many service users may have been involved in other attempts to evaluate or improve services without significant success and may be distrustful of new attempts to do the same. Time, persistence and patience are useful, as well as good community links. Recruitment may take a long time.

Barriers of prejudice and discrimination

Prejudice and discrimination exist in service user groups just as they exist in other communities (Wallcraft *et al.*, 2003). To maximise levels of participation and ensure that everyone can participate fully, especially in a mixed group, clear messages about discriminatory behaviour need to be made, behaviours challenged where needed and safe spaces created where necessary.

Good practice in recruitment

Methods for overcoming the barriers to group recruitment include the following:

❖ Reach out to a range of mental health service user groups, local community and voluntary organisations, advocacy groups, patients' councils and other forums. Visit local day services, housing projects, work projects and other services.

❖ Avoid relying completely on voluntary sector organisations. It is useful to build good links with them at an early stage but they are often over-stretched and 'over-consulted' themselves and may also have good reason to be cautious about a project linked with statutory services.

❖ If you ask people to get involved as interviewers through networks, there is often a snowballing (word-of-mouth) effect over time. As new people get involved as interviewers, news spreads and more people agree to be interviewed and get involved in the project.

❝The networks that people in the group belong to have been really important in establishing credibility for UFM among people who use the service. Word gets around fast.❞

UFM group member

❖ Promote the UFM project through posters in, for example, GP surgeries, social services departments and counselling services. Posters can also be displayed elsewhere, in places where the people you want to recruit will see them: libraries, leisure centres, community cafés, advice centres, and drop-ins. One project placed adverts inside buses.

The recruitment process can often feel a bit 'messy'. It can bring too few people or too many. There may need to be a 'cut-off' point for people joining a project, or it may be a completely open-ended process. For the latter, the capacity to 'fit in' extra training sessions will be needed.

There is still no formal selection process as this has not proved necessary or been seen as desirable in UFM projects. Invite people to join the group on the basis that they are willing to make a commitment to learning, sharing and using skills.

> *The time that I have spent with UFM, meeting all the staff involved from steering groups and the interviewees, has made me a more positive person and has been a very rewarding and enthusiastic experience.*
>
> *Many times I have come home feeling an immense sense of achievement, joy and satisfaction not only on my behalf, but for all those who do the work. It's nice to know that someone, somewhere out there appreciates the work that is being done by people like us. The changes that have come about have been an amalgamation of the efforts of many service users from different walks of life.*
>
> *What I have heard and seen in the interviews is that the same concerns are shared all around in the mental health community. We are all trying to overcome the obstacles that face us and letting staff and other people know what it is really like to be a patient, service user or survivor, whatever you like to call it.*

UFM interviewer

Matching people to tasks

There are a number of ways of being involved in UFM. This makes it possible to match people to different tasks and in this way, allow a wider group of people to be involved (Faulkner, 2004).

It is important at the outset to find out:

❖ what support/training does each person feel they may need? (It will be too late to do anything about this once group training sessions have begun);

❖ what attracted them or persuaded them to take part and what new skills and areas are they interested in?

❖ what level of involvement would people like?

A list can be useful in helping people to think through what their existing skills and interests are and what areas they want to develop through their involvement in the UFM project. Box 7 gives a list of tasks a UFM group will need to carry out.

Box 7: UFM group tasks

❖ producing publicity and posters/drawings;

❖ talking to staff and service users/carers to explain the project;

❖ developing questions;

❖ administration such as typing, phone calls and organising post, etc.;

❖ sampling;

❖ interviewing;

❖ being a companion interviewer;

❖ providing transport;

❖ being available to listen to someone who has done an interview and wants to talk about it;

❖ putting information on to computer;

❖ data analysis (looking at and understanding information collected);

❖ writing the report based on information received;

❖ reading and commenting on report;

❖ meeting with commissioners, etc.;

❖ presenting the findings of report to community groups;

❖ working with/talking to groups of service users;

❖ thinking about ideas to produce changes as a result of the report;

❖ co-ordinating the work:
  • setting up interviews;
  • dealing with petty cash;
  • sending out and writing letters;
  • booking rooms.

UFM projects must be clear about what can be expected from the service users in the group (this can be worked out in a flexible way, on a person-by-person basis and with an explanation of what is on offer to them). Some projects have developed information packs for people who are interested in being involved. Any such pack should not replace contact with the co-ordinator. Contents of the pack could cover the following topics:

❖ what we can offer you and what we expect from you;

❖ information we will need from you;

❖ how would you like to be involved;

❖ payments information;

❖ welfare benefits information;

❖ Inland Revenue (now called HM Revenue & Customs) information;

❖ Licence to practise (see Chapter 7);

❖ Criminal Records Bureau checks;

❖ advance agreement on what happens if you become unwell or in distress;

❖ what to do if you are unhappy or wish to complain;

❖ contract between UFM members and the host organisation.

More information about these topics is provided later in this guide.

Ground rules for groups

To work effectively, you need a culture of equality, mutual support, respect and clear boundaries. The establishment of specific ground rules that are genuinely owned by the group is critical and time should be allowed for this to happen over the first few sessions. There are a number ways to ensure that the group follows the ground rules:

❖ Write them down and hand out copies once there is consensus.

❖ Display them where they will be visible.

❖ If anyone is breaking ground rules, pick them up on this; if this is done from the beginning, it will encourage others to do the same.

❖ Review ground rules regularly: perhaps every three to four months.

❖ Ensure that new members get copies and have a chance to contribute.

Among the essential ground rules are:

❖ confidentiality;

❖ all members to have opportunity to contribute;

❖ respect for difference and for difference of opinion;

❖ one speaker at a time;

❖ everybody is welcome irrespective of sex, race, mental health diagnosis, disability, background and sexuality.

66 *The essence of developing confidence and enabling things for me is to try to create a human and warm environment. We have to make sure that this doesn't get lost.* 99

UFM group member

Forming the group

Early group sessions need to be devoted to clarifying the purpose of the project, establishing the group agreement or ground rules and doing initial work of recruiting and publicising the project. Crucially, this is also the first time some people will have had the opportunity to talk about their own experiences (of having a diagnosis and of services). But when they start to interview others, they will have to be able to separate their own experiences from those of the people they are interviewing.

As with any group, a combination of both large and small group work is useful, depending on how personal the material is that people are being invited to share.

Peer feedback as well as co-ordinator feedback and individual supervision and support can be used as the main mechanism to ensure that people are up to the job and feel comfortable and safe in what they are doing.

> ❝No one can live without hope. That's what being involved with UFM has helped to get back. That's what's been so important and I can see how it has helped others in the group too. Hope that something good can come from all the pain and loss, and hope that my ability to do any serious and valuable work is not over for the rest of my life.❞
>
> UFM group member

Supporting the group

It is always best to establish support processes at an early stage. Although in many ways rewarding, UFM is challenging work. Group members need to know how to get support and it is the co-ordinator's responsibility to actively encourage people to use the supports that are offered.

Support mechanisms should include both peer support and 'buddying' where a more experienced member supports a new recruit (as long as the boundaries and systems are clear), and semi-formal supervision with debriefing by the co-ordinator. Mentoring has not been widely used in UFM projects to date but it, too, is a valuable way of providing people with individual support.

Depending on people's circumstances, other types of externally provided formal or informal support may be appropriate, including information about medication, advocacy, self-help and advice groups and forms of talking therapy. There must be clear boundaries for the co-ordinator, who must not be expected to give this degree of support to people. This can be a difficult balance and, again, is the reason why good supervision and support structures must be in place.

Difficulties that UFM groups have faced

In any group, difficulties can arise; however, they are not regular occurrences in UFM groups by any means and where they have arisen, they have usually been resolved.

Example 1: What to do when a team member is struggling

The co-ordinator should talk with the member about any difficulties they are having and what support could be offered. Taking time out from the project may be an option or perhaps just taking a break from the interviewing. The co-ordinator should make it clear that when the person feels the time is right, they can return to work on the project.

> ❝I think it is important to have discussions with people about these issues at the outset, so that they can say what their warning signs are and you know who to call etc. I think it's helpful to have some kind of process of agreeing that people feel well enough to do interviewing.❞
>
> Former UFM group member (now managing a research project)

Example 2: How to ensure that problems do not arise during the interviews

In one UFM team, an interviewer reported back to the co-ordinator that her colleague had made an inappropriate comment to an interviewee who had disclosed their experience of self-harming. To reduce the risk of this type of problem arising, the co-ordinator should quality-check the work being done by:

❖ observing all group members in interviews from time to time;

❖ organising training so people are used to giving feedback to each other in a constructive way and actively encouraging people to challenge their peers if incidents such as the one described here occur;

❖ continuing training and practice until good boundaries become second nature;

❖ debriefing interviewers after each session;

❖ ensuring that notes are sent to all interviewees inviting them to make contact with the co-ordinator, in confidence, if they feel there has been a problem during the interview.

Example 3: Acknowledging different levels of participation within the group

The co-ordinator should ensure that the group understands that people are likely to participate in different ways and that some will be more able and willing to commit time to the project. Clarify what work has to be done, allowing space for people to take on more or to cut back as circumstances change.

Difficulties may arise when, for example, some people are putting in extra hours, perhaps because they feel responsible for getting the work done, when others are not available because they need some time away. The converse can also be true when people in the group may be ready to take on more but feel they may be taking work away from others.

CHAPTER 5 Training

Many people who come to UFM do so out of a strong desire to see changes in the way mental health services are delivered. Research is seen as a vehicle for highlighting some of the problems that exist and making changes. Few people come to this with research experience. The main aims of the training are threefold:

❖ to identify and develop the skills and experience that people already have and that they can bring to the research;

❖ to increase the confidence of group members in applying these assets to the UFM process;

❖ to provide some basic theoretical knowledge and the opportunity to learn, share and practise necessary skills.

When should training take place?

Often the membership of the UFM group changes in the first few weeks of a new or existing project, as people decide whether the project is for them at this point in time. Remember, this is not uncommon in training of any kind, so try not to be disheartened by these changes or see this process as a waste of time. UFM is an open-ended process, and allowing people to see whether it is right for them has advantages in the longer term; people know about the project, speak of it to others and some may rejoin the group at a later stage.

> *One of the biggest challenges for me so far has been returning to UFM three-and-a-half years after I initially joined (I pushed myself before I was ready). It feels great that I've been able to take part now and has also really helped me to see how far I have come.*
>
> UFM group member

Who should deliver the training?

Ideally the co-ordinator will have experience of both research and training, as well as direct experience of using mental health services. We suggest that the co-ordinator has at least a good understanding, if not experience, of research so that they can successfully support the UFM work. However, the support of an external trainer who can train the group alongside the co-ordinator can be very useful, especially if the co-ordinator is new to training as well or does not have experience of providing training. We would suggest that, given the intense nature of the sessions, there are two trainers for all groups, but definitely for any that are larger than eight or nine people. The co-ordinator should remain responsible for co-ordinating training, with whatever supports are necessary.

Where group members already have research experience from a previous project or from a different source, they also need to be encouraged to share this knowledge and to support the delivery of training to the rest of the group.

External trainers who are recruited for their specific knowledge and skills should preferably also have had experience of the mental health system (see Appendix 3 for a list of service user organisations). Survivor or service user involvement is widely established in many areas and people can be invited to speak on a specific topic just for one session. External service user/survivor trainers could be also be sought independently through recommendation and you may be lucky enough to find service users who work in an academic setting, such as a local university, or from within a trust research department.

Planning the training

We recommend providing some 'core training' at the beginning of the project and supplementing this with extra training at each stage of the project.

When planning the initial training, practical considerations will include:

❖ **Venue:** Find a location that is neutral, away from mental health service sites. Although it is always tempting to use such facilities if they are free of charge, people may feel uncomfortable or unsafe, especially in hospital settings if they have been an inpatient there recently. As with all training, the venue needs to be comfortable, pleasant and accessible, with provision for small group work and refreshments, including lunch.

❖ **Number of sessions:** Typically the core training will run for between six and eight sessions, depending on what is included in the basic training and the amount of time spent developing the questions, although repeat sessions may be necessary and time is needed for practice and piloting.

❖ **Length and frequency of sessions:** Most groups hold weekly meetings. Negotiate times with the group: often the choice is for sessions running from 11 am to 3 pm, to take account of travel difficulties, the needs of people on heavy medication and those with dependants.

❖ **Size of groups:** To some extent this will depend on the size of your project but in general, starting with a group of 10 to 14 is reasonable. Numbers usually fall off after the first couple of sessions, and this often results in a core group of eight to ten people. If the number is greater than this, then it may be difficult to allow enough time for the work to be done and to attend to everyone's needs.

What should the training focus on?

Training and the early stages of the UFM research take place alongside each other. The initial or core training should focus on the basics of service user research. It is important to provide some background information without making it too daunting for the group by giving them too much information. Training also needs to focus on what is often called 'questionnaire design' but in research terms is more accurately known as developing an 'interview schedule'.

For small projects with a very specific focus, the development of the interview schedule can take place within the training session. It can be useful to have each of the group sessions split between training and 'UFM work', or with one 'work session' following a training session.

For more complex projects a start can be made on developing the interview schedule during training, but the full process may take several weeks and training may have to be resumed when this has finished.

Many people will need time to share their stories of using mental health services; this is a necessary part of bringing the group together. It may be the first time they have ever been able to honestly tell others about their experience of services.

However, ultimately, being able to separate their experience from that of people whose stories they are hearing is critical for a 'good' interview to take place. Ensure that there is strong emphasis on good listening skills and on being accepting of other people's views.

The interview techniques require a lot of practice and reinforcement of good listening skills. A mixture of techniques, role-play, brainstorming and even quizzes can be used. New problems may have to be dealt with: in one project, the co-ordinator noticed that one person was struggling in the way she asked the questions and came across as 'flat'. Voice training was arranged to help her and others in their approach to interviewing.

Training should cover the ability to disclose experience appropriately within an interview setting; this is a key component of training. Disclosure will be enough to convey shared experience; for example, disclosure by an interviewer that they have used services locally too. However, nothing should be disclosed that might make the person being interviewed feel that the opinions they wish to express will be judged. Small group work with members observing and feeding back can help to make this clear. If the budget allows, watching a video-recorded interview or even listening to an audio recording is a good way of learning about good interview techniques.

Box 8 gives a suggested core training programme for a UFM project using face-to-face interviews as its main method of collecting information.

Box 8: A suggested core training programme

Part 1: Preparing for the research

Forming the group

❖ Negotiate ground rules within group

❖ Share personal stories

❖ What will happen with the research findings and the services being evaluated?

❖ What relevant skills does the group already have?

What is research?

❖ Importance of evidence

❖ Basics of research – quantitative and qualitative data, the research cycle

Box 8: A suggested core training programme *(continued)*

❖ Different types of interview

❖ Confidentiality and consent

What is UFM?

❖ Why service user researchers?

❖ The aim to implement findings

❖ Brief history of UFM

Part 2: Developing an interview schedule

Focusing

❖ Local relevant issues and personal experiences

❖ Clarifying the focus of the evaluation

What should the schedule look like?

❖ Open and closed questions

❖ Avoiding leading questions

❖ The length of the schedule

❖ Demographic questions (age, gender, etc.)

Drawing up the questions

❖ What have others already done?

❖ Brainstorming questions

❖ Eliminating and refining questions

Part 3: Interview skills

Basic interview skills

❖ Body language

❖ Active listening skills

❖ Plenty of practice in interviewing skills

❖ What not to do!

Interview challenges

❖ Keeping the interviewee on subject

❖ Not influencing the interviewee by relating own experience or views

❖ Supporting distressed or distracted interviewee

❖ Being non-judgemental

Box 8: A suggested core training programme *(continued)*

Other aspects of interviews

❖ Introducing and ending interview

❖ Confidentiality and safety

❖ Roles and responsibilities of interviewers, i.e. boundaries, not counsellors but there to collect information albeit in a supportive and respectful manner

❖ Taking notes

Support for interviewers

❖ Personal support/debriefing

❖ Supporting each other in roles (interviewer and note-taker)

❖ Supporting safety for each other

Practicalities

❖ Payment to interviewee – receipts, when, who, incomplete interviews

❖ Sources of information and help for interviewees

❖ Meeting up before interviews

❖ Support meetings

Training pack

A great deal of information may be generated during training sessions. If time allows, it can be very helpful for group members to have a training pack, which contains summaries of the information that they can use between sessions and before interviews to refresh their knowledge.

The training pack can build on the recruitment information pack. These are some suggestions for the contents of such a training/UFM work pack:

❖ outline of project and flow chart of local service structures and how they fit together;

❖ training programme outline and individual session plans;

❖ ground rules;

❖ beginner's guide to research;

❖ ethical and equalities issues in interviewing;

❖ group communication exercises;

❖ good interview guide and exercises – personal safety/good practice in conducting interviews;

❖ notes on confidentiality and bias;

❖ notes explaining jargon and abbreviations such as CPA, PCT, SHA, CMHT, PICU, etc.;

❖ space for the interviewer's notes and diary pages to encourage them to reflect on how an interview has gone and issues it has raised;

❖ useful telephone numbers.

Further training

It is important to continue looking at other training requirements as the project progresses. This may not be essential to start with if the co-ordinator or others in the project have some of these skills, but it is important to increase the level of skills within the group in the longer term. As well as the obvious benefits to those concerned, it helps to stop the project becoming too reliant on any one individual, which may leave the project vulnerable if and when those individuals move on. Training in the following may be needed at some point:

❖ protocol and project design;

❖ dealing with ethics committees;

❖ data collection and data entry;

❖ data analysis;

❖ report writing;

❖ feedback and dissemination;

❖ presentation skills;

❖ negotiation skills (especially at the implementation stage).

CHAPTER 6

Payments

The UFM process draws on the skills and experience of group members. These skills and experience are highly valuable and this needs to be reflected in appropriate financial reward. At the time of publication, there is renewed debate about the impact that benefits legislation has on the involvement of service users in all kinds of areas, including research and audit. New rules may be proposed to simplify and promote user involvement while the Welfare Reform Bill may also bring about major changes in the benefits system. In practice, this means that the way individuals are financially rewarded or assessed may change quite a bit (DH, 2006b).

It is important to ensure that group members have easy access to expert benefits advice. To this end, it is helpful to develop good working relationships with the following:

❖ an independent welfare rights agency: ask for a named person to take a link role. It may be possible to set up a dedicated work-related advice service for your interviewers, but funding may be needed;

❖ Jobcentre Plus: it may be possible to arrange an outreach service whereby an adviser comes to a meeting. Find out if there is a local customer services liaison officer;

❖ a mental health or care trust: some trusts employ welfare rights advisers. Ensure that the advisers used by your interviewers, wherever they are based, have expertise in issues relating to work and mental health;

❖ HM Revenue and Customs.

We strongly recommend that you obtain up-to-date advice as the regulations change frequently. It is good practice – and also the most simple – to use existing guidelines and policies from official bodies such as HM Revenue and Customs in order to determine, for instance, what level of payment should be made for mileage costs and whether or not this payment is considered to be income. Contacts for further information are listed in Appendix 3.

Box 9: Payment systems for UFM projects

UFM project based in a primary care trust

The group developed the following payments policy:

❖ Each UFM group member received independent welfare rights advice from the local Citizens Advice Bureau to determine hours of work and rates of pay allowed.

❖ UFM interviewers signed a terms and conditions contract and gave bank details for payment.

Box 9: Payment systems for UFM projects *(continued)*

❖ After each meeting/interview, UFM group members completed expenses forms, which were signed off by the project manager.

❖ Payments were made into bank accounts (or occasionally by cheque) from the PCT's UFM budget.

❖ In addition, the project manager liaised with the Department for Work and Pensions to ensure that there was no confusion between UFM and regular work.

UFM project hosted by a voluntary sector organisation

❖ Each UFM member received a UFM pack in which all practical and formal information about their involvement in the project was laid out clearly. This included the policy on payments.

❖ The minimum wage hourly rate was paid for attendance at meetings and for pieces of work (e.g. data entry).

❖ A fixed amount was paid per interview, plus travel expenses if the interview took place away from the office. In this case, travel expenses did not count as income as far as Inland Revenue rules were concerned.

❖ A fixed amount was also paid for presentations to teams and at conferences.

❖ Travel expenses were paid on production of a valid receipt. The project followed the Inland Revenue policy on payments for mileage. It also paid a bicycle mileage rate. When UFM members were paid for their work, reimbursement of travel expenses to the office was regarded as income by the Inland Revenue. Some members therefore opted to be paid travel expenses and not to be paid for the work, while some chose payment for work and not for travel expenses.

❖ Travel expenses were paid in cash, on the day.

❖ All other payments were made by cheque or postal order.

❖ No advance on payments for work was made.

❖ Child-care costs were paid (minimum wage hourly rate) on production of an invoice from the person caring for the child.

7 Criminal Records Bureau checks and honorary contracts

Although Criminal Records Bureau (CRB) checks can sometimes scare off potential UFM members, they have become an established practice with many organisations and employers. UFM does not escape the CRB requirements, although it is important to stress that they do not apply to everyone or for all projects. For further information visit the following websites: www.crb.gov.uk/ and www.disclosures.co.uk.

The requirement for CRB checks is a fairly recent development. The purpose of these checks is to protect groups who fall within the category of 'vulnerable adults'. This group includes people who use mental health services as well as the elderly. Children are covered by a separate check.

A CRB check shows a person's history of spent and unspent criminal convictions, depending on the nature and seriousness of the offence. There are two levels of disclosure, standard and enhanced. The enhanced level is usually required for people working alone with vulnerable adults and children. See the full details on the Criminal Records Bureau's website, www.crb.gov.uk/.

The UFM interviewer is in a position of trust and the requirement to have a CRB check is likely to apply to all those UFM group members who will have direct access to service users contacted and recruited through a trust, a local authority or another organisation such as a charity. In a UFM context, the project co-ordinator and anyone interviewing is likely to need an enhanced check.

While CRB checks are usually seen as a risk assessment tool, they also serve to highlight other issues such as whether an individual has, for instance, a history of committing theft. A risk assessment is then made if the person is working with cash or if they are to be alone at a participant's house, where there could be an opportunity to take money or goods.

It is important to stress that CRB checks are not always required – a risk assessment should be made for each job role. For instance, strictly speaking, since UFM workers always interview in pairs, they may not need a check at all. However, it is probable that the organisation in which they are doing UFM will insist that they undergo a CRB check.

Some UFM members may have come into contact with the criminal justice system, for all kinds of reasons, often when they have been unwell. The idea of having to go through such checks may worry and even alarm some service users to such a degree that they are unlikely to want to go through the process.

However, having a criminal record should not be an automatic cause for employment being refused. Most organisations have an equal opportunities policy and it is up to the employer to consider each case on its own merit. If disclosed convictions come within an area of risk to vulnerable people, a discussion should take place with the individual UFM member with a view to arriving at an appropriate decision. Guidance about the rehabilitation of offenders is available from the National Association for the Care and Resettlement of Offenders (NACRO) as well as from the CRB website.

Disclosure

Clearance from the CRB usually must be obtained before an honorary contract (also known in some areas as a licence to practise) can be granted. A host organisation cannot conduct a CRB check itself. It must go though an umbrella organisation such as the NHS trust with which the project is working.

Anyone applying for CRB clearance must complete an 'application for Disclosure' form. Standard CRB checks usually take at least three to four weeks to be returned. It is possible to apply for a current and valid standard clearance to be upgraded to enhanced. This process is usually quite quick. If a fresh enhanced check (which will check local police records and spent convictions) is required, this process may take quite some time. As the length of time seems to vary considerably across the country, it is strongly advised to apply for Disclosure as soon as possible.

Box 10: Sample UFM CRB policy

The position of a UFM worker is one of trust. UFM workers come into contact with and interview vulnerable people in a variety of settings: in their own homes, in hospitals. Because workers regularly come into contact with vulnerable people they should, like other researchers in similar situations, be subject to Criminal Records Bureau (CRB) checks.

'Enhanced Disclosure' must be obtained from the CRB for all workers. This does not mean that people with criminal records cannot work on UFM projects but each case must be considered on its own merit. If disclosed convictions come within an area of risk to vulnerable adults, this must be discussed with the individual concerned. It may be more appropriate for an individual like this to be involved in the project in some other way. The priority must be to protect potentially vulnerable interviewees.

It is also important to safeguard the privacy of everyone whose CRB check reveals a criminal record. The information that is disclosed should only be seen by:

❖ the UFM research co-ordinator, their manager and other staff within the organisation who need to know;

❖ the local mental health trust if the UFM is carried out in an NHS setting.

This information needs to be stored securely in a locked cabinet. Access to this cabinet must be restricted to appropriate staff. Clear policies should be in place to govern all the procedures connected with CRB checks.

Honorary contracts or licences to practise

Honorary contracts, or licences to practise as they are also sometimes called, are effectively a formal contract of employment between the user researcher and the NHS trust/hospital and deal with the rights and responsibilities of each. Such a contract will need to be secured in order to get access to certain types of information (data) when research is being conducted within an NHS setting, the most obvious of these being contact details of service users or patients. Honorary contracts can be obtained from the personnel department (often called human resources or HR). Some organisations, such as local councils, have their own CRB departments.

Applying for an honorary contract or licence to practise may involve completing occupational health screening forms, and/or attending occupational health interviews, something else that may deter service user interviewers. Liaising with the local occupational health (OH) office at the mental health service is an important step in ensuring that any unnecessary obstacles are removed or minimised early on (see Box 11).

The research and development director of the relevant trust is usually responsible for agreeing honorary contracts but, if not, they will be able to tell you what the procedure is. This can also be your first point of call for getting advice and help with contacting service users and asking them to take part in the research or audit.

Box 11: Occupational health screening

In one project the co-ordinator met with the local occupational health manager early on and talked through the project with them, including how UFM works, the UFM ethos, issues of social inclusion that this type of work promotes, training and, even more importantly for this purpose, the level of supervision on offer to UFM members. Work supervision is given by the co-ordinator and more complex emotional supervision is bought in from a professional counsellor.

This had a very positive outcome and it was decided that it was not necessary for UFM members to go through the occupational health screening or interview process. Insufficient information and communication about this type of research, and about user-led research in general, seems to be the reason why people are put through this stressful process by occupational health departments.

CHAPTER 8

Research design/methods

UFM is different from traditional ways of doing research because it asks questions from the perspective of local service users.

This is partly because questions developed by a UFM project feel more relevant and make more sense to people as they are based on a concrete, grounded understanding of the issues they face on a daily basis (e.g. being slowed down by medication or being admitted as an inpatient and not having a bed or being given any information on admission). It is also because of the relationship between interviewers and participants (based on shared experience as service users), which has been shown to produce more open and honest and therefore more valid responses:

> *Firstly, the questions (developed by service users) tend to cover a much broader range of issues than traditional tools. But even where the topics covered are similar, user groups generate different types of question to those found in professional scales. For instance, professional interviews, like UFM interviews, often ask about medication. But professional interviews tend to focus on issues of compliance whereas UFM groups design questions asking about choice, dignity, information about side effects and respect. UFM questions are also very detailed and specific. UFM groups want to know exactly…what it is about taking medication that users like and do not like.*

(Rose, 2001)

This chapter explains how to design a study and describes the choices available when doing this.

Defining the scope of the research

It is important to be realistic at the planning stage about the scope of the project and identify the specific aspects of a service that the research should focus on.

> *Both projects I've been involved in have grown in scope and ended up with too much data that couldn't be analysed. This is a real waste of effort for everyone.*

UFM Group member

There are a number of questions to be considered when defining the scope of the research. Box 12 shows how the focus of one study on inpatient care was decided.

Box 12: Identifying the focus of a study on inpatient care

❖ What do we already know (from previous local or national research) about inpatient care?

❖ Are we interested in finding out about the inpatient experience of all service users in one hospital or across a number of hospitals?

❖ Are we particularly interested in the experience of a particular community of inpatients, for example, those who have been detained under the Mental Health Act? If so, what aspects of the experiences of this group of people are we interested in?

❖ Do we want to compare experiences of different sub-groups of people detained under the Mental Health Act?

The research area identified was: service users' experiences of three adult acute psychiatric wards. It focused on those who had been discharged from hospital in the previous three months and looked at their experiences of the care programme approach process, relating to admission and treatment, information, ward environment, primary nurse, psychiatrist and discharge planning/ implementation.

It is important that research is clearly focused on what aspects of people's experience you most want to find out about. It is difficult to manage the investigation of too broad a research area. Interviews become too long or too general to cover what is important and to get enough detail. Once you have defined your research area, you need to decide on the method you want to use and on the type of information (data) you want to collect.

The three different methods of data collection

The UFM model usually employs three main ways of gathering information: individual interviews, focus groups and site visits. The UFM team, together with the research supervisor, will need to decide which of these three methods is the most suitable for their study. It may be that combinations of all methods are used or only one.

The research supervisor is external to the project. They ensure that the work is carried out to good research standards and they support the co-ordinator. Where necessary, there may be two supervisors working with the co-ordinator: one who advises on research and the other who gives support on group issues.

Individual interviews

These are called 2:1 interviews because two UFM group members will interview one service user. Usually one person will ask the questions while the other records the answers, usually by writing them down or if necessary by using audio recording equipment or a video camera. The person recording will also help out with prompts if necessary. This type of interview can take between 20 and 75 minutes.

Advantages

❖ Individual interviews allow for the participant to have all the attention focused on them. More detailed information is therefore given. This method is good when the area of research covers issues that some people may find difficult to discuss in a group.

❖ Interviewer(s) usually find them easier to carry out because they are more likely to follow a fairly structured list of questions and as a rule individuals are easier to manage than a group.

Disadvantages

❖ An individual interview can be intimidating, particularly if it is being recorded in some way.

❖ People may find it hard to reflect on their experiences on their own.

❖ 2:1 interviews can be very costly and generate a lot of data.

Focus groups

Focus groups are interviews with small groups of people (6–12 participants). One or two people will be present to encourage a discussion using a set of questions also known as a topic guide. Focus groups are usually tape-recorded and/or extra notes are taken by the co-facilitator who might note, for example, when there was a lot of gesturing or tearfulness. It is important to create a safe atmosphere that enables everyone to participate.

Advantages

❖ The focus group is useful for exploring what, how and why people are thinking in a certain way.

❖ It makes use of shared and diverse experience to stimulate discussion.

❖ It helps to generate more questions (for use in site visits or 2:1 interviews).

❖ Some people feel more comfortable discussing things in a group.

❖ Interactions in the group can prompt comments that may not otherwise have arisen.

Disadvantages

❖ Some people may feel uncomfortable disclosing sensitive aspects of personal experience in a group setting.

❖ It is less easy to conduct a focus group and to ensure that all participants are able to contribute; some people may dominate the process.

In UFM, focus groups can be used as a method in their own right or to generate themes for the development of interview schedules.

Site visits

On site visits, one or two members of the UFM group go on prearranged visits to a site, e.g. an inpatient ward, accompanied by the UFM co-ordinator. The UFM members are shown around the service by a member of staff and spend time talking to any service users who happen to be present who are willing to be interviewed. These discussions may happen on a one-to-one basis or in pairs, and occasionally in small groups. A site visit workbook will be used to note events and the interviewer's impressions and conversations with staff as well as service user comments on sets of questions covering different topic areas (see Appendix 2 for examples).

Advantages

❖ Site visits are a way of getting views that may otherwise be bypassed.

❖ They often provide some flexibility, by making it possible to choose between small group interviews and individual interviews.

❖ They can cover a very broad range of topics.

❖ A site visit gives interviewers an opportunity to observe the environment, e.g. an acute inpatient ward.

Disadvantages

❖ Obtaining the necessary privacy may be difficult.

❖ Information gathered can lack systematic detail.

A UFM project can gather data using one or more of the methods described here. Specific training may be needed to support the method(s) chosen. Which method or methods are chosen will depend to a large extent on the setting and the area to be researched. For example, site visits can be very useful in looking at inpatient experiences. In this case, timing of site visits is important and should not be early in the day when ward rounds are taking place.

66*On one of the site visits to the ward, we saw a woman being forcibly restrained with far too much force and the lead up to this. Details were logged and reported formally to the ward manager but the incident was only referred to more generally in the report for confidentiality reasons.* 99

UFM co-ordinator

Quantitative and qualitative data

Information that is collected through research methods is called data. The data gathered by a UFM project includes quantitative data and qualitative data.

Quantitative data

Quantitative techniques record information numerically. Quantitative data comes from asking closed questions, where users are given a limited set of possible answers. Closed questions allow only yes and no answers (see Figure 2).

Figure 2: Example of a closed question		
	Yes	No
Do you know what the care programme approach is?		

Even things that may not be thought of as quantitative, such as satisfaction, can be assessed by creating a scale to measure them. For example, a scale of 1 to 5 could be used for rating satisfaction where 1 = very unsatisfied, 2 = unsatisfied, 3 = neither satisfied nor unsatisfied, 4 = satisfied and 5 = very satisfied. A rating for 'don't know' could also be included.

Advantages

❖ Data from large numbers of participants can be pooled together.

❖ It may be easier to gather and analyse.

❖ It is easier to code if using computer software.

❖ It is easier to make simple summaries of complex issues.

❖ Service providers like it because it is helpful when presenting overviews.

Disadvantages

❖ Data gained may lack richness and detail.

❖ Individual experiences might be lost.

❖ It provides no way of collecting details about issues that only become clear during the research process.

Qualitative data

Qualitative data records what things mean to people. Qualitative data typically comes from asking open-ended questions to which the answers are not limited by a set of choices or a scale. An example is asking someone to give more details about their response, e.g. "What do you mean when you said you weren't sure about X?"

Other examples of qualitative data include answers to questions such as "How could your care have been improved?" or "What would you like to have been offered instead?" where the response is not restricted to a pre-selected set of answers.

Advantages

❖ The data obtained is rich and detailed.

❖ More detailed information about individual experiences is gained.

Disadvantages

❖ Qualitative data can be more time-consuming to analyse and present.

❖ It may be less respected by service providers and some academics, although recently there has been a shift to a more positive perception of it.

❖ It usually means restricting the number of participants.

Although the two methods may appear contradictory, they can and do in fact complement each other. UFM often uses a combination of both qualitative and quantitative methods, leading to a statistically based report supported and informed by more detailed qualitative information.

It is important to strike the right balance. A good UFM report will avoid relying too heavily on statistical data alone; a huge collection of figures can appear uninformative and hard to 'digest' unless supported by the qualitative data. On the other hand, too many open-ended questions will result in qualitative information that is difficult to collate or analyse and can appear unstructured without the support of quantitative data. Gathering too much qualitative data by obtaining very full personal accounts can also raise ethical questions about having obtained far more information than can be analysed and written up, given the resources available. If you are using quotes, make sure the person quoted cannot be identified.

CHAPTER 9

Developing tools for the research

Once you have decided what research methods are going to be used and what kind of data you want to collect, the research tools such as interview schedules (questionnaires), focus group guides or site visit workbooks need to be developed and tested. This chapter explains these different research tools in more detail and how they can be put together in a UFM project.

Interviews

There are three levels of structure: structured, semi-structured and unstructured.

❖ Structured interviews:

- have a rigid (fixed) design where exactly the same set of questions are used for all participants;

- use closed questions, for instance through tick boxes that allow for a 'Yes, No or Don't know' answer, or rating scales with tick boxes which ask 'To what degree were your needs met?' for a 'Fully, Mainly, Neutral, Not really, Not at all' answer.

❖ Semi-structured interviews:

- use a looser structure;

- use a topic guide or prompts in part (on agreed themes) together with a set of closed questions;

- allow the questions to follow the flow of the interview in order to ensure that all the topics are covered.

❖ Open (unstructured) interviews:

- enable the participant to lead the interview, which becomes an in-depth investigation of their background, experiences and feelings;

- can evolve from one participant to the next, so questions may vary between one interview and another.

Most UFM projects use a semi-structured interview format. This is because it allows more qualitative information to be gathered than is possible with a structured format, but is quicker and easier to administer and analyse than an open interview. Interviews usually begin with a series of closed questions, followed by open questions that ask for more detailed answers or comments about that particular question. For instance: "How many times did you see your GP at times of crisis?" might be followed by an open question about the actual experience of seeing the GP, for example, "How did the GP respond to your crisis?"

Questions (whether open or closed) that 'lead' to a response of a certain kind must be avoided (e.g. "How much disturbance is there on the ward?").

Focus groups

Focus groups can make use of various techniques/tools such as imaginary case studies, a topic guide (e.g. "What was your experience of going to Accident & Emergency like?"), probing questions (e.g. "Can you tell me a bit more about...?") and follow-up questions (e.g. "You mentioned earlier that... What was most upsetting for you, X or Y?").

Sometimes, the methods will be determined by practical considerations:

> ❝*Due to the large number of very different services involved in our review, it was decided that carrying out a set of site visits and discussion [focus] groups would be the best method. To carry out one-to-one interviews across all services would have involved interviewing a huge number of users which was beyond the scope of the current review.*❞
>
> Quote from a UFM report (1998)

Site visits

The tool for site visits is called the workbook. A workbook is set out differently from a questionnaire because it records information that is obtained from more than one source. (A sample page from a workbook is shown in Appendix 2.)

The workbook consists of sets of questions covering different topic areas. For example, in the case of inpatient site visits, topics covered have included treatment and medication, facilities and activities available and leave arrangements (some site visit workbooks have had up to 30 topic areas).

Each topic has a page within the workbook with the question prompt at the top. On the remainder of the page there are sections for noting:

❖ **the source of evidence**, e.g. service user or staff comment or observation by the UFM visitor;

❖ **the evidence itself**, i.e. what was actually said or observed;

❖ **recommendations** that are made by service users, staff or the UFM visitor;

❖ **a rating** given by the UFM visitor on a scale from 1 to 5 for each topic area/question, based on what has been said and observed.

Developing the questions

Whatever method is used for collecting data, the research questions are created by the UFM group during or following basic training.

The process normally starts with a group discussion about the subject area. This often begins with personal reflections by the group on their direct experiences. Topic areas (and questions) can also be identified through outreach work. This could take the form of meeting with other service user groups or carrying out preliminary (unstructured) interviews with other people who have experienced mental health services or who have a mental health diagnosis other than those who are 'represented' within the group.

Headings from interview schedules produced by other UFM projects on the same subject area may be useful as a checklist for overlooked topics, although this should not be a substitute for the group going through the question development process. What is relevant to ask may differ according to how particular issue(s) are being experienced in a local area.

Box 13: Developing questions

In the case of the first UFM project in Kensington & Chelsea and Westminster, when developing the site visits questionnaire for inpatient service users, the group discussed and explored their own experiences of inpatient services to produce an account of a 'day in the life' of an inpatient. From this they developed a comprehensive list of all the issues that should feature in the questionnaire. The co-ordinator then produced this as a list of questions in the first draft of the questionnaire. (Extract from Rose *et al.*, 1998)

The next stage is to work the topic areas/headings into themes and, from these, specific core questions are formed. It is usually the job of the project co-ordinator to distil the UFM group's work into a first draft of the interview schedule/site visit workbook or focus group guide. This and further drafts will then be taken back to the group for comments and reworking. It may need to be redrafted several times before the group feels it is ready for use but it has the advantage that the group becomes familiar with the questions and can refine them accordingly. Box 14 gives ideas for how an interview schedule might be structured. To make the schedule easy to navigate it should be easily readable and marked clearly (e.g. with arrows) where sections can be 'skipped' if they are not relevant to the person being interviewed. A similar format can be used for a focus group guide or site visit workbook.

Box 14: An interview schedule structure

Introduction

❖ Introduce the project and the interviewers.

❖ Explain the process (breaks, how long the interview will take, whether there is any payment).

❖ Reassure people that what they say is confidential and that they don't have to answer every question.

❖ If the interview is recorded, double-check that the participant is still happy with this.

❖ Explain what type of information is being sought.

❖ Describe what will happen to the findings and allow time for any questions.

❖ Depending on whether ethical approval is needed, get consent forms signed if this has not happened already.

❖ Ask if the interviewee is comfortable and ready to begin.

Warm-up questions

Ask simple questions to ease participants gently into the interview, e.g. about types of services used and for how long.

Box 14: An interview schedule structure *(continued)*

Main body of questions

The schedule needs to have a structure that will help the interview 'flow' well. The layout needs to be clear and easy for interviewers to use. This will save time and avoid unnecessary explanations and repetition. Prompts are helpful in directing interviewers to a different part of the document, e.g. 'if answered "No", go to question 15'.

Demographic information

These questions help to 'close down' the interview formally. They may include age, gender, ethnicity, employment/marital status, etc. These are important questions that will help to give a broad description of the people who have participated in the research and allow you to break down responses by some of these characteristics: e.g. you may find that a particular group of people were having more problems with a particular issue. Interviewees should be allowed to define their own ethnicity, where possible from the classification used by local service providers.

Closing comments

These generally include questions about how people have experienced the interview and how they wish to receive feedback about the project.

Detachable information sheet

Include a detachable pull-out sheet of local and national organisations, addresses and phone numbers at the end of your questionnaire. One of the most common UFM research project findings is that people feel they do not have enough information about sources of support and advice about a whole range of subjects.

Piloting the tools

All research tools should be piloted before starting the interviews. This is the opportunity to find out how well the questions flow, fit together and, most importantly, whether they make sense. Decisions about the final length and balance of open and closed questions can be made at this time. Also the group can check if all the issues agreed on at the planning stage have been covered.

The tools need to be piloted with people other than the UFM group members, to gain a fresh perspective on them. Ideally, they need to be piloted with a group of people similar to those you want to interview in the main study. Planning the pilot interviews at the same time as you are working on the interview schedule is usually helpful.

Reliability and validity

Reliability and validity are ways of measuring the quality of a research tool.

Reliability

This is the degree to which a research tool is consistent and reproduces the same results, independent of the circumstances. These might include which interviewers are conducting the interviews (this is called inter-rater reliability) or whether interviews are taking place at different points of time (test-retest reliability).

We suggest only one of the various reliability tests is necessary (inter-rater reliability). Since a UFM project has more than one interviewer, check whether different interviewers are carrying out and completing the questionnaire or workbook in the same way. Each interviewer should fill in a schedule and later an independent person can calculate the degree of agreement in their records: which should be at least 75%.

Validity

This describes the degree to which research measures what it is supposed to measure. A research tool (e.g. questionnaire) may be reliable but it may be measuring something completely different from what was intended. For example, questions may measure 'friendship with other patients' rather than the overall experience of hospital which is the intention of the research project.

There are different ways of measuring validity:

❖ **Face validity:** "At first glance, does the tool appear to be assessing the desired qualities (e.g. satisfaction with services)?"

❖ **Content validity:** "Does the tool sample all the relevant or important content or domains (e.g. does each question measure satisfaction)?"

❖ **Construct validity:** "Is overall satisfaction with services shown to be firmly associated with responses to individual questions in the schedule?"

CHAPTER 10 Sampling and carrying out interviews

This chapter describes the process for deciding which people will be asked to take part in an interview and how they will be invited.

Sampling

It is important to be realistic at the planning stage about the scope of the project. You cannot talk to all, or even most, of the people connected with the subject you have decided on. Therefore, the people you interview will need to be selected in some way. This is called sampling.

It is important to be clear about how you sample. You will need to be able to show that you have made an effort to ensure that the selection of people is representative of everyone who might have been included (for example all the inpatients in a ward, or all service users of a community mental health service), and not biased in any way. For example, the sample would usually include people from some of the following groups: men and women, people of different age groups, and people from different ethnic groups, unless your research is just focusing on the experiences of a very specific subgroup, e.g. South Asian young men.

Random sampling

Random sampling is a method of selecting your participants in a way in which every member of the population has an equal chance of being selected. Random sampling ensures that bias is not introduced regarding who is included in the survey.

In previous UFM projects participants have been randomly selected from lists of current service users provided by the local trust; often these are lists provided by a trust's clinical audit department. Random sampling allows for a wide range of service users to be given an opportunity to have their say. In this way it is hoped that those who are more isolated, and perhaps less mobile or confident, will be given a chance to express their views, in addition to those who are more willing or able to attend service user groups or service planning meetings.

However, there may be times when random sampling is not appropriate or necessary. This is because a project purposely looks for a particular section of the population, for example those who have (or have not) used crisis services. This is called convenience or purposive sampling and has been used in UFM projects.

The UFM model usually employs random sampling to select the participants when conducting one-to-one interviews. However, for site visits and focus groups the interviews take place with self-selecting participants.

It is much better to randomly select a smaller number of people and work hard at achieving a high response rate than to randomly select a large number with the hope that at least a certain proportion of them will agree to be interviewed. A higher response rate will mean a more representative sample.

> **Box 15: A simple random sampling technique**
>
> Each name on the caseload of a community mental health team is given a number, between one and 500. One hundred numbers are randomly generated. The people with these numbers are then approached to be interviewed.

Statistical significance

A research finding is said to be statistically significant if it can be said with confidence that the result could not have been arrived at purely by chance. Statistical tests can be used to say how confidently this can be stated. In the case of UFM, this means being confident that the findings from the sample can be applied to all the users of the service. This means having a sample that is big enough to generalise with confidence but small enough to be manageable for the project group.

Barriers to sampling

Service user records are not easily accessible

Sometimes the information about service users of a team/service may not be accessible because records are not kept electronically or are not up-to-date. This can create serious delays. Currently, under the Data Protection Act, even with a licence to practise, access to medical notes and records is restricted and ethical approval is given under strict conditions. The Central Office for Research and Ethics Committees (COREC: www.corec.org.uk), as well as the local NHS Research and Development Support Units may be able to advise on this delicate aspect of the process.

Staff involvement

Generally staff involvement in sampling, recruiting and/or introduction of service users should be kept to a minimum. Being monitored or evaluated by service users may be perceived by some service providers and staff as intrusive and controlling.

> 66*Among service providers, it is not yet readily appreciated that mental health problems do not necessarily preclude service users from having rational balanced views about the services that they receive. Although such a perspective is now rare in the research literature, it appeared to be still evident among some frontline staff.*99
>
> ex-UFM co-ordinator

Where participants have been selected by staff, it is important to take care that people have neither been put under pressure to participate nor unduly discouraged.

Introducing the project at an early stage to sector and team managers will engage staff in the process and makes communication easier if and when problems arise. Keeping them updated about progress is important too.

Concerns are often raised by staff about the prospect of face-to-face contact between service users in an interview setting, most commonly expressed in terms of whether such contact is 'safe or appropriate', whether people being interviewed are well enough and whether boundaries will be maintained.

Addressing staff concerns about the interviews is crucial to the success of any UFM project, and it is important to build on the commitment and awareness that does already exist among staff.

> *As mental health workers, we must recognise the major change in culture and practice that is necessary if the power of service users to determine the shape and content of services is to increase. This change involves:*
>
> ❖ *A shift from secrecy to openness and sharing of knowledge and information*
>
> ❖ *Acceptance of the limitations of our skills and the value of the expertise of personal experience*
>
> ❖ *Recognition that some of the things we do, however well intentioned, may be harmful*
>
> ❖ *Willingness to listen and learn from those whom we serve*
>
> ❖ *An ability to reflect on our practice and change what we do.*

(Perkins & Repper, 2003)

Carrying out the interviews

This section provides advice about how to conduct the interview itself. Appendix 1 also gives further guidance on carrying out interviews, safety issues and confidentiality.

Choosing the interviewer

If possible, give a choice of interviewers to the participant. Making assumptions about gender and ethnicity is dangerous, so always ask the participant if they have any preferences. Interviewers may also have preferences, e.g. a woman might prefer not to interview men and vice versa, although this should not lead to discrimination against any particular group of people.

Service users in the group should not interview people at services they currently attend or have received recently. This experience can be personally difficult and it is also advisable that they do not interview people they already know, as this can affect the quality/outcome of the interview.

Using interpreters

It is usually difficult, not to say expensive, to use professional interpreters. For this reason, if there is a need for translation, it may be a good idea to check the funding organisation's arrangements for providing interpreters, as it may well be possible for the UFM project to make use of this service. Many NHS trusts have access to on-site interpreters, in particular in larger cities.

Owing to the nature of UFM interviews, it is important that the interpreter be made aware of the remit of their role in the context of research. It can happen that the interpreter relates only part of what the participant is expressing or effectively changes what the person is trying to say. Ideally, a professional interpreter would be used or one of the interviewers would speak the language of the participant.

Interviewing in pairs

It is good practice for all UFM interviews to be conducted in pairs. This has the advantages of:

❖ addressing safety and peer support needs;

❖ ensuring someone is there to take notes/ensure equipment is working and keep an eye on the time;

❖ enabling the person asking the questions to fully concentrate on the interview and their interaction with the interviewee;

❖ allowing the recorded data to be compared and inter-rater reliability (consistency) to be established. Both interviewers need to complete the interview schedule.

Finding the right location

Service users may sometimes find it difficult to go out: therefore their home can be a practical and safe choice for them to be interviewed in. Don't assume that this will be the case, however. As with any interview, safety issues for the interviewers need to be considered. Also, many unexpected interruptions can occur, e.g. relatives can walk in and out of the room or want to sit in on the interview.

Public places such as cafes should be avoided as venues for interviews. They may feel relaxed and convivial but they lack privacy, and could therefore affect confidentiality, and they can be noisy.

Mental health facilities, e.g. a day service or ward, can provide a good location, but bear in mind that participants may not feel comfortable being in a service setting. In this case the confidentiality of the project needs to be stressed. A room within a neutral place, e.g. a voluntary sector organisation, is another alternative. Where possible, give participants a choice.

Health and safety issues

These are as much about the interviewers' as about the interviewee's welfare, if and when difficult situations arise during the interview. It is therefore advisable to:

❖ work in pairs (as discussed previously);

❖ ensure that the co-ordinator knows where and when someone is going out to do an interview;

❖ carry a mobile phone so that one of the interviewers can contact the co-ordinator or someone else agreed in advance, should they encounter a serious difficulty at the interview;

❖ agree in advance a way of communicating concerns about the location of or the circumstance surrounding an interview (e.g. if one of interviewers feels threatened or there is a sense of danger, or if one of the interviewers feels unable to cope or is distressed). This could be an agreed message (e.g. "I have a headache");

❖ let the co-ordinator know when the interview is completed.

Ensuring confidentiality

Confidentiality can be assisted by allocating a number and the initials of the interviewer to the completed interview schedule. The information sheet given to participants should also clearly mention whether recording equipment will be used so that they can make up their mind about this in advance. It is important to check, prior to starting the interview, whether they are still happy to be recorded, as they have a right to change their mind at that point.

It is important to explain where and how the interview schedule, tapes from interviews, etc. will be stored and who has access to this data. Emphasise that the information collated in the final report will not identify participants. Be explicit about circumstances in which an interviewer would breach an interviewee's confidentiality, e.g. if they talked about harming themselves or other people. Most research ethics committees expect this to be included in the information for participants.

Debriefing

Interviewers should discuss any issues that arose during each interview. This might be about disclosure of sensitive information that needs to be dealt with by the co-ordinator or by an outside agency (e.g. regarding child protection). It may also be that an interview has touched a bit too closely on the interviewer's personal experience and caused them distress.

Debriefing can be done as a group or individually. It is an important form of supervision and it must not be neglected. However, it is also important to have a system by which external professional emotional support can be obtained, free of charge to the UFM worker; for example, should those issues reach beyond the scope of the UFM co-ordinator's supervision abilities and remit, or if an interviewer requires it because they are feeling burnt out or overwhelmed.

Accurate recording

A key role of the UFM interviewer is to ensure that information is accurately and properly recorded. For instance:

❖ Use legible handwriting.

❖ Quote participants verbatim in the notes. If the interviewer is unsure about a quote or comment they have written, they should check with the participant (perhaps at the end of the interview) whether what they have written is accurate. Weeks and months sometimes may go by before the team has time to analyse the data and it will then be too late to contact the interviewee for clarification.

❖ Avoid using shorthand terms and expressions that cannot be understood by other members of the team.

❖ If video or audio tapes are being used, there should be a budget for transcription.

If recording, it is important to explain the recording technique to the participant and seek their informed consent. Some people may find this inhibiting. In the case of taped interviews, the quality of the transcript will be important and it is essential to get an experienced person to do this work.

Conducting site visits

It is essential to set up the visit in advance with the unit manager and select a day to attend when service users are likely to be available (e.g. not on a ward round day or during a popular activity). It is helpful to send some posters and information about the UFM project to be displayed on the site in advance to advertise the visit.

The ideal number of site visitors is four, including the co-ordinator. It is important to ensure that there is a mixed group of interviewers for site visits. On arrival, it is usual for the site visitors to request a tour of the unit with the manager, who can answer questions as they go. The site visitors can then disperse around the site and spend the rest of the visit speaking to any service users present who agree to be interviewed.

The site visit interview follows a semi-structured format. For this reason and to avoid an off-putting professional appearance, the site visitors do not usually bring the workbook to the site. Instead, they carry a 'prompt card' (a small laminated card listing the questions that can be referred to unobtrusively) and a small notebook to record responses. Issues of confidentiality still apply here.

Site visits usually last for two hours or so and each site visitor may conduct several interviews. The visit should be followed by an immediate debrief – perhaps just a shared discussion in a coffee shop on the way home. Some site visitors like to begin filling in the workbook at the debriefing, especially if the co-ordinator's support is being requested.

Practical obstacles that may arise include:

❖ staff deciding who can and can't be interviewed;

❖ language (where there is a need for an interpreter);

❖ venue (this may be noisy or there may be a lack of privacy).

Objectivity, bias and reflexivity

Traditionally, the view among those who fund research into mental health is that it should be rigorously 'scientific' and free of judgements or opinions of any kind. This has created a hierarchy in research. For instance, randomised controlled trials (RCTs – large-scale research testing a hypothesis or a type of treatment) are deemed the 'best' research studies, the so-called 'gold standard', because they are seen to be more objective and therefore more valid. Most of these studies have been professionally controlled and, by virtue of this, what is important to service users rarely figures highly in them. This situation is beginning to change and service users continue to campaign hard for further change.

In recent years, mental health trusts and universities have begun to involve service users in research projects. This is partly an effect of the requirement for applicants for NHS research funding to involve service users (and carers). Although progress is patchy, there are good examples, such as the Service User Research Enterprise (SURE), based at the Institute of Psychiatry.

UFM is one of the strands of user-led research that seeks to counter the status quo and to value people's experience of using mental health services as highly significant, valid and 'expert'.

At some point during the UFM project, however, there may be accusations of bias. Research led by service users is often challenged in this way (Turner & Beresford, 2005).

Objectivity and bias

Objectivity is still often seen as an important aim in social science research and frequently it is an attempt to mirror the approach of the exact sciences. UFM has sometimes been criticised for not providing 'valid' results as there are not enough guarantees of objectivity. The belief that service user projects may be biased towards producing a negative picture of the services that are being evaluated still prevails in the minds of many. However, it is widely accepted by social researchers that all social research (whether it is done by more traditional researchers or by user researchers) is, by its very nature, biased. The research agenda and the values of the person conducting the research will always have an effect on the research findings.

Given that bias is impossible to avoid in any piece of social research, it is important to be explicit about how it is affecting the research. This does not make the research invalid. On the contrary, bias in UFM is a valuable and positive element. This is because it starts from a different place, that of experience, which encompasses a focus on people, their feelings and situations.

It is inevitable that both the approach taken by the researcher and any power differentials that exist between them and the interviewee will affect the information that is elicited. Where interviews are conducted by service users, the power differential is reduced.

UFM provides some objectivity by structuring the research process, training researchers and checking both reliability and validity. Some projects have been able to compare their findings with those of more traditional research.

An example of this is a finding from one UFM report which showed that a high percentage of psychiatric inpatients did not know who their key worker was (Bristol Mind, 2002). A year later, a trust audit on the same issue produced the same figure.

Reflexivity

The influence of the researchers themselves on findings has long been recognised in qualitative research. An important way of addressing these influences is to gather "sufficient detail on the way the evidence is produced for the credibility of the research to be assessed" (Shipman, 1988). This is known as reflexivity.

Reflexivity has become a very important part of social research, in particular when dealing with life stories and narrative research. It has come about as a realisation that the social researcher can no longer be considered an independent or neutral party, simply collecting data and not having any effect on the interview process or on the participants.

In the delicate relationship between the researcher and the researched, it is important to be clear that the choices and assumptions that researchers make affect how the voices of the participants are translated. Reflexivity in UFM then becomes a tool to develop awareness of what other biases, such as personal beliefs and expectations, may be present, in particular during interviews or data analysis. Supervision, research diaries and group discussion are aids to reflexive practice.

CHAPTER 12

Analysing data

Once the interviews are complete, there will probably be a great deal of information to analyse. One of the key criteria for UFM is that findings are examined by service users. If the co-ordinator and the research supervisor are not service users, they should not carry out the analysis on their own.

The group can at an early stage discuss their impressions about the types of themes that they feel have been emerging. Interviewers may also be able to draw on their notes to remind them of things that may have had particular meaning for them. This is all part of the reflexive process.

People from the group often get involved in data inputting in the chosen software package, and training should be made available, as early as possible in the project, to facilitate this process.

While statistics and themes emerge from the analysis and should be shared and discussed with the group, the actual written analysis for the report should be done by a much smaller group of people (realistically only one, two or three), usually the co-ordinator plus interviewers and/or the research supervisor when needed. This is really for practical purposes, as individuals have different styles and ways of writing. It is also helpful if someone looks at the data and the write-up who has a little distance from the interviews; preferably a service user, who could be the research supervisor. They can take back to the group drafts of the findings section of the report, with their comments.

It is important that the findings are described and presented and a discussion held about what these mean, using the unique perspectives of all service users involved in the UFM group, including the co-ordinator. This is a core aspect of all service user-led research. In some research projects, the results of UFM interviews have been analysed and written up entirely by professional researchers. This is not 'true' UFM.

> **❝** *I found the process of interviewing extremely humbling. As interviewers, we were entrusted with very precious objects, namely the participants' testimonies and experiences; these had to be treated with proper care. Another notable challenge came during the analysis and writing up of the report. I found it difficult to go along blindly with some aspects of the external advice we were given, which was pushing for a far more statistical approach to the findings that, to my mind, was too remote from what had been shared with us. My personal instinct was to go for something more qualitative, thus interpreting the information from our perspective as service users. I feel that using people's feelings and experiences as evidence is as appropriate and relevant as statistics.* **❞**

UFM interviewer

Collating and storing the data

A good system is needed for securely storing all the data that has been collected. Written information needs to be kept in locked cupboards. Storage of video and audio recordings should follow strict rules in order to preserve confidentiality. The data needs to be stored to allow later access, should participants feel their testimony was not represented fairly or to check the validity of claims made in the report. The Data Protection Act is quite clear. Local trusts may have data protection officers who will be happy to answer any queries. The research and development (R&D) support units can also help. Here are some of the basic ground rules for the storage of this type of raw material:

❖ Recorded material on cassette tape must be stored in a locked cabinet and only accessed by the team for the duration of the project. Ensure that labels only bear the interviewee's identity number and no name. Those which are sent away for transcribing should be sent securely and the transcriber should agree to abide by confidentiality rules (by signing a document to this effect). Once the project is completed, the tapes should be stored in the same manner for a period of five years and then destroyed.

❖ With digitally recorded material, computer files should be password-protected for the duration of the life of the project. Saved audio files should be erased from the recorder after each interview. Anonymised and password-protected interviews saved on CD-ROMs should be sent for transcription by post. If files are sent over the internet for transcribing, an encryption method should be used. Once the project is over, the audio files should then be transferred onto CD-ROMs and stored for five years, after which they should be erased.

Enter quantitative data on to a computer as it comes in. This both avoids being overwhelmed later in the process and makes it possible to pick up on and check any discrepancies with interviewers before too much time elapses. Data that will be used for analysis needs to be stored separately from any personal information that has to be stored. Access to both sets of data needs to be restricted in order to ensure confidentiality. Personal information such as names and addresses should not be stored any longer than is absolutely necessary and should not, under any circumstances, be used for anything other than contacting participants about the research, and then only in ways that they have agreed to.

Analysing quantitative data

Using suitable computer software is essential for collating, processing and presenting quantitative findings. There are two types of software that can be used for this. These are spreadsheets (such as Excel) and specialised statistical analysis software (such as SPSS).

For most UFM projects, spreadsheet software should adequately address the needs for analysing and presenting data. This software is normally cheaper than statistical analysis software. It is also more likely that there will members of the group who are already familiar with using it.

Specialised statistical software does provide opportunities for data analysis that are not available with spreadsheets. For most UFM projects this advanced level of analysis will not be required, however. Making use of these possibilities requires not only familiarity with the software but also a more thorough knowledge of advanced statistical methods.

Although most software does contain in-built tutorials, it is recommended that members of the team who are involved in data entry and/or analysis receive adequate training before they start. Allow sufficient time for people to become familiar and competent to input data accurately. Regularly check that data input is accurate.

Analysis of the data as it is presented in UFM reports often concentrates on proportional analysis. This can be done by stating the frequencies or the percentage of people who are satisfied or dissatisfied with a particular aspect of a service.

Correlations may also be presented; these show how strongly two particular factors are related. For example, a report may show that one group of participants has different experiences from those of the rest of the sample.

Analysing qualitative data

The way qualitative data is used can range from obtaining quotes and descriptions that support the quantitative data to a systematic attempt to discover underlying themes and ideas.

Thematic analysis seeks to describe the different themes that emerge from the data. As the name implies, this involves going through the data to find instances where things have a similar meaning or refer to the same thing. Each time the themes can be regrouped and redefined to arrive at a limited but comprehensive number of categories.

Adequate and thorough training is needed if qualitative analysis is going to be done correctly. When this does happen the qualitative analysis of the data can involve many members of the group and become a focus for lively discussions between them about the findings. This kind of analysis can be a very in-depth procedure, involving complex analyses of all the qualitative data that has been gathered.

66 *Before the software was used, we as a group discussed what important themes had emerged from the qualitative aspects of the interviews. Once all the data had been put into the software package, we again as a group refined these themes into categories. We then took the data home and counted how often these categories came up.* 99

UFM researcher

For more in-depth advice on qualitative research, refer to the *DIY Guide to Survivor Research* (Mental Health Foundation, 1999).

CHAPTER 13 The final report

A printed report ensures that the findings are easily available long after the completion of the project. There have often been significant problems at this stage of the process for some UFM projects.

❝*On completion of all 30 interviews, it became obvious that the group was not going to be involved in the writing of the report; instead it was being written at the university. While this was happening, the UFM group had to keep pushing to be kept informed of any progress, and to have any involvement in its contents. Eventually, we were allowed a minimal input and some alterations were agreed.*❞

UFM co-ordinator

Other projects have been so under-funded that they have been unable to produce a final report and have been apprehensive about asking for more funding for fear of jeopardising future projects.

While one of the most obvious and important ways of distributing findings is in the form of written reports, the report should be part of a wider plan for disseminating the findings (see Chapter 14).

Other projects have made a point of ensuring that all interviewees can receive a report if they wish, and that reports are distributed widely to other service user groups as well as to relevant statutory and voluntary sector staff. Some projects have produced two forms of report: a full report, containing all the relevant information and data, and an 'executive' summary, which is more accessible and focuses on providing other service users with the main findings and conclusions. We know of one project that produced more than two reports. The Bristol UFM report *Crisis…What Crisis?* (Bristol Mind, 2004) covered a wide range of services and a number of different executive summaries were produced, aimed at specific teams and services.

Effective reports describe the research process fully and openly, including an explanation of how being service users has influenced the report. In presenting the findings, group them in clear and logical categories (not necessarily following the different sections of the questionnaire), and show how the findings are based on what was said in the interviews (as opposed to just expressing the views of the group). Produce understandable and concise conclusions and recommendations. A clear, well-laid-out report will reflect a clearly constructed argument.

Clear and accessible language is important. The report is not only aimed at commissioners and other researchers; it will also be read by participants and the service user community, who may not have experience of the research process, the services that are being talked about or the kind of language used in services and research.

In presenting the findings it is important to get a good balance between presenting quantitative and qualitative data. Illustrating themes from the data with quotes can be very powerful and mean that many service users can recognise experiences similar to their own in print. This can have a big impact, for example on service users who felt they were the only ones with certain experiences or feelings.

A graphic representation of your findings (e.g. a graph or bar chart) can make them more accessible to readers; however, including too many in the main body of the text can make the report less readable.

Use colours, fonts and features that can be photocopied without losing quality and large enough to be accessible by people with visual impairments or learning disabilities. The report should have an authoritative layout and design. It need not be boring but should reflect the quality of the work that has gone into it. It is important to remember that the aim of the report is to reflect the collective experience of service users in a concise and understandable way so that it can be used for guiding changes to services.

Structuring the report

It is important that reports are structured clearly. Box 16 gives a checklist of items to include.

Box 16: Report checklist

❖ Title page including UFM project logo and date

❖ List of names of members of the research group

❖ Table of contents

❖ Acknowledgements and any disclaimers on policies of local authority, trusts, etc

❖ Glossary of abbreviations and terms

❖ Executive summary: a short version of the findings aimed at people who don't have the time or the inclination to read the full report. It has to be concise and clear enough to convey the most important messages

❖ Introduction to the UFM model and to the project

❖ Methodology: a description of the process used to produce the information presented in the report

❖ Results: a presentation of the main findings from the research

❖ Discussion: a description of what the findings say about the service being researched

❖ Conclusions: the group's summary of what the findings mean

❖ Recommendations: what should be done to address the project's findings

❖ References: other publications quoted in the report

❖ Appendices: additional information including findings not covered in the main body of the text; copies or summaries of the interview schedule; personal accounts of interviewers; feedback from participants; contact details for project; list of resources.

Previous UFM reports can act as a guide to how the report can be presented. Information on these can be found on the UFM network website (www.ufmnetwork.org.uk).

CHAPTER 14

Dissemination, implementation and outcomes

> "If we are to increase equity, the biggest challenge is to improve the quality of services available to everyone."

(Perkins, 2003)

Service users repeatedly emphasise the importance of improving services as a primary motivation for becoming engaged in research. Research methods like UFM are therefore inherently attractive in that they hold out the promise for change.

Dissemination and implementation are about ensuring that the research influences the way services are run and are thus an essential component of the project. It is also important and ethical to show other service users not only that their experiences have been heard but also what has been achieved and what other action is planned (Turner & Beresford, 2005; Faulkner, 2004). Yet this work is often perceived as more challenging than the research itself.

Many UFM projects in the past have only received enough funding to conduct the research. Some have not even had the money to print copies of their final report.

This chapter shows how projects can be disseminated effectively.

Presentations

Presentations are an important way of disseminating findings, especially to other service users. For many service users and other interested communities of people, attending a presentation is a far more accessible way of hearing about the research than reading a report and it gives them the opportunity to ask questions and debate the issues raised. Presentations also offer new people the opportunity to get involved in taking forward the report's findings or in planning the next research project.

Overheads or projected computer presentations can be very effective, as some people find it easier to take in information visually and for most people visual information complements what they hear. Presentations need careful planning in order to decide what the main messages are and to select the information that will support these. It can be very easy to present too much information.

Some members within the group may already have the skills to make effective presentations and be able to share their knowledge with others. But training is still useful to develop skills further and ensure that there are more people in the group who are able to do this.

Presenting findings is not a one-off process: UFM groups often continue to present the findings for up to 18 months after the conclusion of the research. This should be considered when negotiating funding. Budgets for presentations should include the costs of:

❖ training

❖ advertising

- ❖ equipment
- ❖ travel
- ❖ reimbursements for time
- ❖ location
- ❖ refreshments.

An event to launch the final report may also be used to publicise the project and recruit group members for the next project.

Newsletters and websites

Brief summaries of the report can also be reproduced in newsletters that are sent out in mailings by other service user organisations and in mailings to staff. This is an effective way of ensuring that there is widespread knowledge of the work that has been done. Community venues, including libraries, are also good places to leave summaries.

Some projects have made their reports available on their own website or elsewhere on the internet, and some trusts have put their UFM reports on the trust website. Online access to these reports has been invaluable to other service user groups seeking to undertake similar projects. It is also a way of making service user led research more visible to a wider public.

We are not aware of projects that have used the local press or other media to disseminate their findings, but there is the potential to reach wider audiences in this way.

Audiences

Effective dissemination should focus on three main target audiences: service users; local service providers and commissioners; and the wider public.

Service users, as researchers and as interviewees, invest a large amount of their collective time in UFM research, (for little or no payment) hoping for change. When the final report is not disseminated effectively, it can confirm the belief that their views and experiences are unimportant and irrelevant to service providers. Service users report having been asked about their experiences during other service evaluations and audits, but having not heard anything afterwards and having not seen any changes. It is important that service users, especially service users who have contributed to the project as interviewees, or otherwise, are able to obtain free copies of the report.

Dissemination should extend as far as possible within the services that have been evaluated: from frontline and support staff to board and management levels and including other agencies such as housing providers, voluntary sector organisations, churches, other health services, including Accident & Emergency, and the police.

It is also important to present the findings to commissioners. Not only is it important that they are aware of service users' experiences of the services they commission; these presentations are an opportunity to persuade commissioners that UFM should be a regular part of their monitoring and evaluation of services.

Some staff may have research experience and are likely to scrutinise the data and the findings more closely. There is therefore a need to ensure that the members involved in presenting the report have a good grasp of the data and findings and are correctly prepared to argue those appropriately. After all, that too is part of the research process experience.

Disseminating the findings of UFM research to a broader audience has not had much emphasis to date. There have been publications such as *Users' Voices* which have looked broadly at UFM findings across the early projects (Rose, 2001) but there is also a lot of good work that is only known locally.

Wider dissemination is needed, and projects that have sufficient funding could think about ways of disseminating their work, for example, through presentations at conferences and articles in journals. The UFM Network has begun to pool knowledge and experience by linking projects with each other, making a list of UFM reports available on the internet, developing guidelines for UFM research (UFM Network, 2003) and contributing to this publication (for more information see www.ufmnetwork.org. uk). There are also other service user research and involvement forums such as Shaping our Lives, the Service User Research Group England (SURGE) and the Mental Health Foundation's online research network, the Service User Research Enterprise (SURE) and the Survivor Researcher Network. Website addresses are available in the resource guide in Appendix 3.

Implementation

If UFM is to be effective, service providers must seek to make changes based on the recommendations developed from the report findings. Experiences of implementation have varied enormously. Sometimes the report alone may be enough to stimulate change. Often more active participation by service users in the process of change can ensure that the findings have more impact and that this is publicised.

Creating or adapting effective structures is very important. Active service user participation in using UFM findings as a catalyst for change can take a number of forms. These include the following:

❖ The UFM report is used by other user groups as part of their ongoing work to influence services.

❖ An action plan is drawn up by UFM project members and service providers, with the latter overseeing the implementation.

❖ An existing forum of service users and service providers adopts an action plan that is developed from the UFM report.

❖ A new forum of service users, service providers and commissioners is established specifically to implement the findings from a UFM report.

It is important for UFM groups to plan ahead for this stage of the work. Often it can make all the difference to have the support of one or two members of staff in reasonably influential positions. An effective strategy for implementing changes involves prioritising the desired changes according to their level of importance, and to the likelihood of them being achieved. Even apparently simple changes can take a distressingly long time to implement and it is important to maintain motivation by focusing on achievable goals.

Identify the staff who should be involved in this process. Management support can be important, but it is also important to involve practitioners themselves to effect change in the way they work. Adopting a 'two-pronged approach' involves working with senior managers who can champion the recommendations at a strategic and policy level, and with frontline staff who can make real changes to practice. It is important to keep some members of the UFM project involved in the implementation process as they are familiar with the research and know what questions and findings have led to the conclusions and recommendations.

It is also important to involve other service users and user groups whenever possible. These groups have often spent years campaigning on the same issues. People involved in these groups are also aware of where barriers to change have been encountered previously. In fact, it has been possible with some UFM projects to begin to overcome barriers that have been, or seemed, insurmountable. This may simply be due to the fact that the timing is better or that the same message coming from a research base has a greater impact.

Outcomes

Many UFM projects have reported positive changes to services. These range from cultural changes, e.g. a more general spirit of collaboration between staff and service user groups, to specific changes in the way services are provided.

Often it remains difficult to discern how many of these changes are due to the UFM process and how many are due to a combination of the UFM work, the efforts of other user groups and staff initiatives.

Projects with the long-term funding to repeat their research at regular intervals (e.g. annually) can provide excellent initial baselines to gauge if and how services are improving. For example, the Kensington & Chelsea and Westminster UFM project has been able to show a year-on-year improvement in service users' knowledge of the care programme approach (CPA) (Rose *et al.*, 1998).

Box 17 gives some examples of how UFM projects have worked to ensure that their findings were implemented.

Box 17: Outcomes

Project 1: Acute inpatient care

This UFM project looked at the experiences of service users in acute inpatient services. After the report was produced an action group was established which was co-chaired by the UFM co-ordinator and the clinical nursing lead of the mental health trust. This group had an open membership and included people from other service user groups. For one piece of work a sub-group was set up to look at ways to improve admission procedures. Initially they focused on the two main hospitals in the study but it became clear that their work was applicable to the wider trust. This resulted in revised procedures, a patient handbook written collaboratively by staff and service users, and training to support the implementation of these new procedures.

Project 2: Housing needs

This project looked at the needs of service users from the Supporting People housing support programme as part of a wider review by a local authority. The research established people's priorities, which included life skills, security, medication issues and meaningful activity. These priorities were then used by the funders to create good practice criteria for providers of sheltered and supported housing for people with mental health problems.

Project 3: Care programme approach

This UFM project established a steering group chaired by the director of service development at a primary care trust (PCT) with representatives from the UFM team and senior staff at the mental health trust, other PCTs and local authorities. Its remit was to promote and champion the UFM work and findings and to develop and monitor action plans to address recommendations. This contributed to the revision of the mental health trust's policy on the care programme approach (CPA) and led to the development of new policies and practices such as a pre-meetings checklist for staff to complete with service users.

CHAPTER 15

Future directions

UFM has come far since the first project looked at the care programme approach to mental health care in the former Kensington & Chelsea and Westminster Health Authority (Rose *et al.*, 1998). The successes of many of the projects, and the difficulties that have been faced, have developed the model further. At the time of writing, the number of true UFM projects has not been mapped.

For each project that has successfully got off the ground and continued, there are many that have not survived, i.e. either not been funded at all or have not made it beyond a one-year pilot, sometimes despite the most vigorous battles to secure ongoing funding after successfully completing the initial project. This demonstrates how sustainability and funding remain such huge barriers.

Future development

Within the basic model there is still much room for development, especially in relation to implementation and outcome measures. In-depth work on these areas is being done by projects such as SURE but there are many other challenges that still need to be tackled. These future challenges include the following:

Working with new groups such as older people and young people

There are examples of young people being involved in the evaluation of their experiences in care settings, although this is not an area that any UFM projects have yet covered. Extending UFM to services for older people would need the active involvement of those with dementia. People with dementia have already been involved in collectively addressing concerns about services (Cantley, Woodhouse & Smith, 2005), proving that having dementia does not necessarily preclude involvement. But to do this effectively will require training and support for the whole group. Interviews may need to be conducted in radically different ways if they are to be effective.

Working in new service areas, such as forensic services or in prisons and young offender institutions

There is still little user involvement in forensic mental health services generally, despite examples of some very active and engaged user groups in a few locations. Staff are therefore not likely to have experience of actively engaging with user initiatives to improve services. Despite these difficulties, the need for UFM in secure services and prisons is great and the benefits may be considerable.

> *That there is a need for UFM within forensic services seems clear. The coercive nature of these services forces service users to become particularly astute in providing service auditors and other professionals with a distorted picture of services based on service users' perceptions of the answers that are expected. Daily life in forensic services trains service users to provide the answers that are expected, to the extent that this becomes second nature; 'playing the game'.*
>
> (Banongo *et al.*, 2005)

Carer- and family-focused monitoring

Early attempts show that the UFM process might need to be adapted to cater for differing group expectations and needs.

Developing alternative service models

There could be opportunities for UFM to do more work that looks at service users' experiences and need for support beyond what existing services can offer. One way of doing this is through UFM projects that focus on problems that service users face rather than on evaluating one particular service. Provided UFM principles are upheld, an approach looking at gaps and alternative services does have the potential to make change on a broader scale, especially if it feeds more directly into commissioning bodies rather than service providers. Achieving this will mean that people in UFM groups are more involved in strategic planning and commissioning as well as service development.

Exploring new developments in methodology, e.g. participatory appraisal techniques

Participatory appraisal techniques are increasingly influential in the study of community needs (Rose, 2001; Shah *et al.*, 1999). This approach is now being integrated into project plans for some UFM projects that are currently under development. Participatory appraisal techniques in this context involve service users defining priorities for research at the outset in an engaging and enjoyable format which encourages a sense of group purpose and ownership of the project.

Participatory tools (Shah *et al.*, 1999) include using ranking exercises and flow diagrams on flip charts. They can be used, for instance, to identify key aspects of services that people would like to be monitored.

The systematic evaluation of UFM itself as a process and its impact

Funding for this has been sought but has not so far been successful. Such an evaluation needs to be at the very least a true collaboration between service users and others, if not user-led. There has been some evaluation of consumer involvement more generally (Barnard *et al.*, 2005) which has shown that service users were successful in finding ways to change services, based on research findings.

Using modern media

A video project could be used to gather qualitative data and prepare the ground for a UFM project; or video or other media based evaluations could be integrated with and used to adapt a UFM project. This might help to involve people who would otherwise not participate in reports using written media.

Other areas that existing projects are hoping to explore in the future include evaluating services from a Black and minority ethnic (BME) perspective with a BME-only group, evaluating service users' experiences of primary care and looking at the experiences of people with mental health problems who avoid contact with mental health services.

The UFM Network

The UFM Network was formally established in 2003 and has met quarterly since then. Its aim is to:

❖ ensure that the integrity of the UFM model is maintained and adhered to (see the criteria set out in Chapter 1);

❖ provide a safe and supportive space for co-ordinators and UFM group members to share their work and learn from each other.

The Network is open to co-ordinators of UFM projects and members of UFM groups, and some former co-ordinators continue to actively support the Network. As this publication marks the completion of the UFM programme of work at the Sainsbury Centre for Mental Health, co-ordination of the Network will be shared between projects. The Network is not currently funded and will continue to work as a collective.

This guide and the document *Doing it for Real* (UFM Network, 2003) were written by members of the Network.

The UFM Network is not, at the time of writing, a formally constituted group.

If you are interested in getting involved in the Network, or want to get information on UFM reports, then contact the Network through its website (www.ufmnetwork.org.uk).

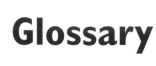

Glossary

Advisory groups

These provide practical help and support to a research project but do not have any management responsibilities. They can be made up of people external to the project, such as professional researchers/academics with a particular interest in the subject, R&D personnel, clinical audit personnel, service users and carers. A UFM project may choose to have an advisory group rather than a steering group, thus leaving the management process entirely to the group.

Advocacy/advocate

An advocate assists a service user in accessing comprehensive, impartial information to enable them to make an informed decision. They may also accompany a service user to a meeting, and represent their views to other people. Advocates are trained and experienced people, often themselves users or ex-users of mental health services, working voluntarily or as paid workers.

Care plan

Each service user should have a personalised care plan which gives details of services to be provided.

Care programme approach

The system by which each person who uses mental health services has their needs assessed and through which plans are made to meet these.

Carer

Carers may be a parent, spouse, partner, child, relative or friend who provides regular and substantial unpaid care to someone who has mental health problems.

Clinical audit

The examination or review of a practice, process or performance in a systematic way to establish the extent to which they meet predetermined criteria.

Community mental health teams

These provide services for people with severe mental health problems outside hospital. They are made up of relevant professionals including nurses and social workers overseeing a defined geographical area.

Criminal Records Bureau

This is a national body in charge of reducing the risk of abuse by ensuring that those who are unsuitable are not able to work with children and vulnerable adults. In order to do this it runs checks on individuals on behalf of employers and other organisations.

Data

Another name for findings, the information collected through research.

Data Protection Act (1998)

Enables individuals to access information of which they are the subject, e.g. their own medical records. It also ensures that data collected through research is properly and securely managed and stored.

Dissemination

The means by which the results of research are given to all the stakeholders (participants, funders, health professionals, carers, user and carer groups, academics and other interested parties). Methods include: written reports, newsletters, presentations, conferences, media, journal articles and the internet.

Equal opportunities policy

A descriptive term for policies intended to give equal access to an environment or benefits, especially to social groups that might have suffered from discrimination.

Evaluation

Carrying out research to judge the value of a service or treatment, usually by making a comparison.

Focus group

A number of individuals gathered together for research purposes because of their experiences and opinions on a particular subject. The members may come from a cross section of the public or a specific section of the population.

Forensic mental health services

Specialist services for people who are in or have been through the criminal justice system and who experience severe mental ill health. The aim is to prevent re-offending among ex-prisoners, persistent offenders and young people.

Honorary contracts

Honorary contracts are forms of contract between a person wishing to undertake research in an NHS setting and that setting. (Also known in some areas as licences to practise.)

Incapacity-based benefits

These are welfare benefits such as incapacity benefit (or IB) and income support (IS) for people too ill to work. IB and IS will be replaced by an employment and support allowance from 2008 for new claimants with disabilities, if the Welfare Reform Bill is adopted by Parliament.

Inpatient

A person who stays in a psychiatric hospital, either on a voluntary basis or who is detained under the Mental Health Act.

Inter-rater reliability (between interviewers)

The measure by which it is possible to check whether both interviewers at an interview have heard and understood the same thing; this ensures consistency in the findings.

Licence to practise

Another term for honorary contract.

Mental health trust

The statutory body funded to deliver specialist mental health care in a particular area. It manages mental health services in the community and hospital.

Mentoring

A process by which a more experienced person (the mentor) assists someone less experienced by giving advice, support and encouragement and acting as a role model.

Methodology

This describes the research process in an ordered and structured way. Its purpose is to illustrate in detail: the background to a piece of research, how it is planned, how it will be conducted, how participants will be recruited, how the data will be collected and analysed, issues of data protection and ethics, how the results of the research will be disseminated and any implementation process.

Primary care trust

A local NHS organisation responsible for the provision of primary care and the commissioning, administration and performance management of health care within a defined geographical area.

Prompts

Prompts are potential questions that could be asked during an interview. They are normally used for semi-structured and qualitative interviews. They serve as reminders of areas and particular topics for the interviewer to explore.

Research and development (R&D)

Each NHS trust has an R&D department. They have a crucial role to play in the approval process of any piece of research taking place in an NHS setting.

Research ethics committees

There are 155 of these bodies in the UK. Their role is to assess proposed pieces of research and to ensure that proper research codes are respected. Health research ethics committees are made up of health professionals, academics, lay members and sometimes service users. The national organisation is the Central Office for Research Ethics Committees (COREC).

Research instruments/tools

The tools used in research to gather data and other information, including questionnaires.

Research process

The means by which any research is developed and progressed from defining the research area and questions to the dissemination and implementation stages.

Schedule

A research questionnaire.

Service-level agreement

A formal contract between different parties, for instance, between a PCT and a user organisation about the funding and the running of a UFM project by the latter.

Steering groups

Some research projects are effectively managed through a steering group. Their function, as the name implies, is to ensure that the project keeps to its aims and objectives and timescales. Like advisory groups they can be made up of a variety of people external to the project, such as professional researchers/academics, R&D personnel, clinical audit personnel, service users and carers.

Supporting People

A government programme that deals with the funding and planning of housing-related support services in an individual's home. It funds, for example, staff based in hostels for homeless people and support workers in group homes. The aim of the programme is to assist people to continue to live independently and, where possible, to progress to a more independent lifestyle.

Topic guide

A flexible set of questions in the shape of prompts which guide the interviewer through an interview or focus group meeting.

User-controlled research

User-controlled research is a reaction to more traditional forms of research which ignored the issues of certain disempowered groups, including mental health service users.

User-led research

This term describes research that is led by service users. Its use has sometimes been criticised for not being clear about the exact nature or level of involvement of service users in that process. It is also sometimes used interchangeably with user-controlled research, although there are differences between the two terms.

Voluntary sector

The voluntary sector is sometimes called the third sector, after the public and private sectors. Voluntary sector organisations are often registered as charities, which operate on a non-profit-making basis, to provide help and support. They may be local or national, and they may employ staff, or depend entirely on volunteers.

Abstract

Abbreviations

ACT	acute care forum
AOT	assertive outreach team
BME	Black and minority ethnic
BMJ	British Medical Journal
CAB	Citizens Advice Bureau
CAMHS	children and adolescent mental health service
CMHT	community mental health team
COREC	Central Office for Research Ethics Committees
CPA	care programme approach
CPN	community psychiatric nurse
CRB	Criminal Records Bureau
CSIP	Care Services Improvement Partnership
DH	Department of Health
DDA	Disability Discrimination Act (1995)
DPA	Data Protection Act
HR	human resources
LREC	local research ethics committee
LIT	local implementation team
MHA	Mental Health Act
MHAC	Mental Health Act Commission
MHF	Mental Health Foundation
MHRN	Mental Health Research Network
NACRO	National Association for the Care and Resettlement of Offenders
NHS	National Health Service
NICE	National Institute for Health and Clinical Excellence
NIMHE	National Institute for Mental Health England

NSF	National Service Framework
OH	occupational health
OT	occupational therapist
PALS	patient advice and liaison service
PCT	primary care trust
PICU	psychiatric intensive care unit
R&D	research and development
SCMH	The Sainsbury Centre for Mental Health
SHA	strategic health authority
SLA	service-level agreement
SRN	Survivor Researcher Network
SURE	Service User Research Enterprise
SURGE	Service User Research Group England
UFM	user-focused monitoring

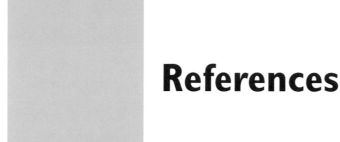

References

Banongo, E., Davies, J., Godin, P., Thompson, J.B. *et al.* (2005) *Engaging service users in the evaluation and development of forensic mental health care services.* London: City University.

Barnard, A., Carter, M., Britten, N., *et al.* (2005) *An evaluation of consumer involvement in the London Primary Care Studies Programme.* Eastleigh: Involve.

Beresford, P. (2005) Developing the theoretical base for service user/survivor-led research and equal involvement in research. *Epidemiologia e Psichiatria Sociale (EPS),* **14** (1) 4-9.

Bowling, A. (2000) *Research Methods in Health.* Buckingham: Open University Press.

Bristol Mind (2002) *User-focused Study of Inpatient Services in Three Bristol Hospitals.* Bristol: Mind.

Bristol Mind (2004) *Crisis…What crisis? The experience of being in a crisis in Bristol.* Bristol: Mind.

Brown, D.G. (1998) Foulkes Basic Law of Group Dynamics: Abnormality, injustice and the renewal of ethics. *Group Analysis,* **31,** 391-419.

Cantley, C., Woodhouse, J. & Smith, M. (2005) Listen to us: Involving people with Dementia in planning and developing services. Newcastle upon Tyne: Dementia North, Northumbria University.

CSIP/NIMHE (2006) *Ten High Impact Changes for Mental Health Services.* London: Care Services Improvement Partnership.

Department of Environment, Transport and the Regions (1998) *Modern Local Government in touch with the people.* London: The Stationery Office.

Department of Health (1998a) *A First Class Service: Quality in the New NHS.* London: DH.

Department of Health (1998b) *Modernising Mental Health Services: Safe, Sound and Supportive.* London: DH.

Department of Health (1999) *National Service Framework for Mental Health: Modern Standards and Service Models.* London: DH.

Department of Health (2000) *The NHS Plan: a plan for investment, a plan for reform.* London: DH.

Department of Health (2003) *Developing choice, responsiveness and equity in health and social care: A national consultation exercise.* London: DH.

Department of Health (2005a) *Creating a Patient-led NHS: Delivering the NHS Improvement Plan.* London: DH.

Department of Health (2005b) *Delivering race equality in mental health care: An action plan for reform inside and outside services and the Government's response to the Independent inquiry into the death of David Bennett.* London: DH.

Department of Health (2006a) *Best Research for Best Health.* London: DH.

Department of Health (2006b) *Reward and Recognition: The principles and practice of service user payment and reimbursement in health and social care*. London: DH.

Faulkner, A. (2004) *The ethics of survivor research – guidelines for the ethical conduct of research carried out by mental health service users and survivors*. York: Joseph Rowntree Foundation.

Faulkner, A. & Morris, B. (2003) *User Involvement in Forensic Mental Health Research and Development*. Liverpool: NHS National Programme on Forensic Mental Health Research and Development.

Fernando, S. (2003) *Cultural Diversity, Mental Health and Psychiatry: The Struggle against Racism*. Hove & New York: Brunner-Routledge.

Ferns, P. (2003) *Letting through Light: Ealing Service Users' Audit*. Rare Sense Ltd. in association with West London Mental Health NHS Trust.

Ferns, P. & Trivedi, P. (2002) *Letting through Light: Service User Audit for North Birmingham Mental Health Trust*. Rare Sense Ltd. in association with North Birmingham Mental Health Trust.

HASCAS (2005) *Making a real difference: Strengthening service user and carer involvement*. Leeds: NIMHE.

Lockwood, S. (2004) 'Evidence of Me' in evidence based medicine? *British Medical Journal*, **328** 1033-1035.

Mckie *et al.* (2002) *The evaluation journey: an evaluation resource pack for community groups*. Edinburgh: Action on Smoking and Health Scotland.

Mental Health Foundation (1999) *The DIY Guide to Survivor Research: Everything you always wanted to know about survivor-led research but were afraid to ask*. London: Mental Health Foundation.

Mental Health Foundation (2003) *Surviving user-led research: Reflections on supporting user-led research projects*. London: Mental Health Foundation.

Oliver, M. (1992) Changing the social relations of research production. *Disability, Handicap and Society*, **7**, 83-87.

Patel, N. (1999) *Getting the evidence: guidelines for ethical mental health research involving issues of 'race', ethnicity and culture*. London: Mind/Transcultural Psychiatry Society.

Perkins, R. (2003) Choice and equity. *Openmind*, **122**, July–August.

Perkins, R. & Repper, J. (2003) *Social Inclusion and Recovery: A Model for Mental Health Practice*. Oxford: Bailliere-Tindale.

Pilgrim, D. (2005) Protest and Co-option – The voice of mental health service users. In: Bell, A. & Lindley, P. (eds) *Beyond the Water Towers: The unfinished revolution in mental health services 1985-2005*. London: The Sainsbury Centre for Mental Health.

Robson, C. (2002) *Real World Research: A Resource for Social Scientists and Practitioner-researchers* (2nd edition). Massachusetts: Blackwell.

Rose, D. (2001) *Users' Voices: The perspectives of mental health service users on community and hospital care*. London: The Sainsbury Centre for Mental Health.

Rose, D., Ford, R., Lindley, P., Gawith, L. & The KCW Mental Health Monitoring Users' Group (1998) *In Our Experience: User Focused Monitoring of Mental Health Services in Kensington & Chelsea and Westminster Health Authority.* London: The Sainsbury Centre for Mental Health.

Rose, D., Fleischmann, P., Tonkiss, F., Campbell, P. & Wykes, T. (2002) *User and Carer Involvement in Change Management in a Mental Health Context: Review of the Literature.* Report to the National Co-ordinating Centre for NHS Service Delivery and Organisation R&D.

Rose, D., Wykes, T., Leese, M., Bindman, J. & Fleischmann, P. (2003) Patients' perspectives on electroconvulsive therapy: systematic review. *British Medical Journal,* **326,** 1363-6.

SCMH (2002) *Breaking the Circles of Fear: A review of the relationship between mental health services and African and Caribbean communities.* London: The Sainsbury Centre for Mental Health.

SCMH (2006) *Policy Paper 6: The Costs of Race Inequality.* London: The Sainsbury Centre for Mental Health.

Shaw, J. (2002) *Expert Paper: Prison healthcare.* National R&D programme on forensic mental health. Liverpool: Liverpool University.

Shipman, M.D. (1988) *The Limitations of Social Research.* (3rd edition) London: Longman.

Shah, M.K., Kambou, S.D., & Monahan, B. (1999) *Embracing Participation in Development: Wisdom from the Field.* Atlanta: CARE. Available from: www.care.org/programs/health.reproductive_health.asp

SURGE (2005) *Guidance for Good Practice – Service User Involvement in the UK Mental Health Research Network.* London: Service User Research Group England. Available from: www.mhrn.info/dnn

Thornicroft, G. & Tansella, M. (2005) Growing recognition of the importance of service user involvement in mental health service planning and evaluation. *Epidemiologia e Psichiatria Sociale,* **14,** (1) 1-3.

Trivedi, P. (2001) Never Again. *Openmind,* **110,** July–August.

Trivedi, P. *et al.* (2002) Let The Tiger Roar... *Mental Health Today,* August, 31-33.

Trivedi, P. & Keating, F. (2006) Personal communication.

Turner, M. & Beresford, P. (2005) *User Controlled Research: Its meanings and potential.* Shaping Our Lives and the Centre for Citizen Participation, Brunel University. Eastleigh: Involve.

User-Focused Monitoring Network (2003) *Doing It for Real: A guide to setting up and undertaking a User-Focused Monitoring (UFM) project.* London: The Sainsbury Centre for Mental Health. Unpublished. Available from www.scmh.org.uk and www.ufmnetwork.org.uk

Wade, D. T. (2005) Ethics, audit and research: all shades of grey. *British Medical Journal,* **330,** 468.

Wallcraft, J., Read, J. & Sweeney, A. (2003) *On Our Own Terms: Users and survivors of mental health services working together for support and change.* London: The Sainsbury Centre for Mental Health/ The User Survey Steering Group.

Williams, J. & Keating, F. (2005) Social Inequalities and Mental Health – An integrative approach. In: Bell, A. & Lindley, P. (eds) *Beyond the Water Towers: The unfinished revolution in mental health services 1985-2005.* London: The Sainsbury Centre for Mental Health.

Wright, P., Turner, C., Clay, D. & Mills, H. (2006) *Practice guide 6: Involving children and young people in developing social care.* London: Social Care Institute for Excellence.

Guidelines

1. Guidelines for carrying out interviews

Prearranged interviews

Introduction

❖ Tell the interviewee your name and that of your colleague.

❖ Thank them for taking part.

❖ Ask them what they would like you to call them.

❖ Tell them that you receive or have received services too.

❖ Remind them of payment and confidentiality.

❖ Remind them they can have a break when they want/refreshments.

❖ Give directions to bathroom if applicable.

❖ Smile, be friendly and be as relaxed as possible.

Location and room layout

❖ Is the room temperature okay?

❖ Bear in mind how and where to position yourself (sit close enough to hear and have eye contact) – position yourself near the door/at an angle.

Introducing the project

❖ Tell them why you are here to interview them.

❖ Check that they are still happy to be interviewed.

❖ Tell them how long the interview will probably take.

❖ Ask them if they have any questions prior to beginning the interview.

❖ Have information available for them, e.g. on advocacy.

Approaching people for interviews 'cold'

On a site visit interviewers usually have to approach prospective interviewees. It is important for interviewers not to disrupt the ward or to cause distress to patients. Here are some tips for approaching patients in addition to following general principles:

❖ Do not approach those who appear visibly distressed.

❖ Do not interrupt conversations.

❖ Emphasise payment/confidentiality/independence/that you are a service user too.

NB: It is useful to publicise your visit a couple of weeks beforehand. If your research involves being at a particular site for several weeks, then people may well begin to approach you.

Before/during the interview

❖ Ensure that someone (e.g. the co-ordinator) knows that the interview is taking place.

❖ Wear clean but casual clothes.

❖ Give the interviewee plenty of 'space' and time to answer questions – do not rush them – be patient.

❖ Make them feel that you are interested in them and their answers – really listen to what they are saying – do not simply read the questions.

❖ As far as possible be aware of how comfortable or uncomfortable they might be feeling.

❖ Make them comfortable by chatting informally between asking the questions.

❖ Take time so you can be calm and in control during the interview.

❖ Speak clearly.

❖ Be aware of your body language, which should be 'open', at ease.

❖ Make eye contact but be sensitive to how much eye contact the person is comfortable with.

❖ Check with the interviewee that any notes you are making accurately reflect what they are saying.

❖ If they appear to be distracted: ask them if they are alright or whether they would like a break.

❖ If they appear to be distressed: acknowledge how they are feeling and offer them a break.

❖ Avoid 'interviewer bias', i.e. saying anything that might make the interviewee change their response to please you or to fit in with your views. Remember that it is important not to express your opinions about mental health services during the interview.

❖ If someone asks for personal information you will need to decide how much to share. If they ask for your address/to meet up, tell them that you cannot. If you feel unsafe/threatened, then close the interview.

Ending the interview

❖ Thank them for participating.

❖ Ask them if they want to read through what you have written down, or would like you to read it back to them?

❖ Restate that their answers will be anonymous, i.e. their name is not on the questionnaire and that their comments will not be identifiable in the report.

❖ Explain what will happen to the interview findings. Tell them about the report/report summary that will be sent to them and any launch event. Say that they are welcome to contact the project if they wish to give further feedback or want to know more.

❖ Give them their payment in an envelope which will already have their name written on it and ask them to sign a receipt. The demographic information and receipt may be combined since they will be kept separately from the research data.

2. Guidelines (checklist) on roles and responsibilities of an interviewer

What an interviewer should do	What an interviewer should not do
Listen for any views about what was positive and what was not good, and for views of how things could have been better.	Make assumptions about what the interviewee would like to say and suggest answers.
Explain the whole process including who you are, your role as a service user interviewer, and confidentiality.	Tell them what to do, e.g. recommend changes for their care.
Encourage interviewee to express what they really feel/think by putting them at their ease.	Give strong opinions on their experiences/talk about your own experiences.
Focus on recording the interviewee's views fully.	Give your phone number or address.
Give them a sheet of useful numbers for access to help/advice.	Accept gifts or offer to come and visit the interviewee to help them with problems
Ring co-ordinator if uncomfortable or not feeling well.	Turn up in a state unfit to conduct an interview, e.g. having had too much to drink.

3. Guidelines for safety

Safety guidelines need to be in place for interviewers, especially when interviews take place in service users' homes. Some suggestions for the content of these guidelines are set out here. It should be noted, however, that these guidelines are intended for dealing with the most extreme situations, and the thousands of UFM interviews that have taken place have never, to our knowledge, resulted in a situation in which interviewers or interviewees have been in any physical danger.

❖ Interviews should take place, wherever possible, during office hours on Monday to Friday. The UFM co-ordinator must be informed of any interviews taking place outside the hours of 9.30 am to 5.30 pm.

❖ Before leaving to go to an interview the researchers must ensure that the co-ordinator has all the details of where the interview is taking place, the name and contact details of the participant, and when the researchers can be expected to return. A simple form with all the details can be used routinely for this.

❖ If interviewers are travelling separately to an interview address, then the first person should wait for the other before entering the premises.

❖ UFM interviewers should be able to contact the co-ordinator or to be contacted in return. The project could consider investing in a couple of basic pay-as-you-go mobile phones for this purpose.

❖ Interviewers can elect to have the co-ordinator call them, five or ten minutes into an interview. Code words or phrases can be used to ask the co-ordinator to:

- call back again after an agreed time;
- call the local police station and ask for an officer to visit the interview address.

❖ During these telephone conversations the co-ordinator should endeavour to ascertain what the situation is by asking questions that can be answered with 'yes' or 'no'.

❖ After the meeting the interviewers should contact the co-ordinator at a prearranged time to confirm that the meeting has been completed safely.

❖ Interviewers should never attend interviews alone, but should always work in pairs.

❖ The pair should agree a code phrase or word between them in order to communicate if one of them feels unsafe and would like to leave.

❖ Mobile phones must be carried at all times and be switched on (silent) during interviews. Workers should familiarise themselves with the number for making emergency calls and set up a 'one-touch' routine on their handset.

❖ The co-ordinator should meet or have a telephone conversation with interviewers at the end of each day to receive feedback.

If things go wrong

If an interviewer fails to report back as arranged, the member of staff expecting to be contacted must immediately:

❖ Ring their mobile phone to ascertain that they are safe.

❖ If necessary, call the local police station and ask for an officer to visit the interview address.

4. Guidelines for confidentiality

What is confidentiality?

Confidentiality is about not giving away personal or private facts about people to others who have no need or right to know them. Interviews within UFM are conducted 'in confidence'; what interviewees say should not be passed on to any other person in a way that would allow them to be identified. Similarly, in discussions within the group, things that people may choose to reveal about themselves or others must not be discussed outside the group.

Why is confidentiality important?

Everyone has a right to have their privacy respected. Many of us will have had the experience of having had details of our private lives discussed openly in meetings and similar settings and will know how unpleasant that can feel. People will only be open and honest if they are sure it is safe to be so. This means that if they criticise people they must know that those people will not be told about it.

What is 'confidential within the team'?

Although confidentiality is vital for UFM to work, it is important to remember that many things can and should be discussed *within* the team. You may have found some of the things that someone you were interviewing told you to be worrying or upsetting. You need to be able to talk about this with colleagues so they can support you and you can support them.

When can we break confidentiality?

There are circumstances where the 'duty of confidentiality' is less important than other things, primarily where there is a definite threat to someone's health or safety. It is possible that UFM workers will come across a situation where they are concerned about how someone has appeared to them or by something they have seen in the course of an interview.

Or you may be aware that another member of the group is finding things very difficult but has chosen not to discuss the problems they are having. These issues should be raised with the project co-ordinator. In very serious cases it may be necessary to decide to break the confidentiality that has been promised. If you do, always offer a full and frank account of the reasons why it was felt necessary to do so as soon as possible to the person affected.

The information that is kept

Personal data such as name and contact details may need to be kept in case an interviewee needs to be re-contacted. This data should not be kept any longer than necessary and should be kept separately from the research data itself. Both sets of data need to be stored securely in compliance with the Data Protection Act.

A good source of information about confidentiality and other ethical issues is *The Ethics of Survivor Research* (Faulkner, 2004).

5. Guidelines for setting up advisory/steering groups

Draft terms of reference

Members of UFM project steering groups and advisory groups should be selected on the basis of their knowledge and understanding of the principles of UFM work, and also for their connections in the locality where the work is taking place. They can be a mixture of service users, professional staff from mental health, social or voluntary sector services, and individuals with particular relevant expertise, for example in research.

Steering groups and advisory groups have some roles in common, and others which are particularly to do with either steering the project, or advising the project team. A UFM co-ordinator and their team can define what role they want the group to play in their project, and draw up their own terms of reference. The following is a guide to what might be included.

Steering groups and advisory groups

Their role is to:

❖ develop and promote the project and model in accordance with UFM principles set out in this guide and *Doing it for Real* (UFM Network, 2003);

❖ support and advise the UFM co-ordinator and UFM team on planning and carrying out and disseminating a UFM project;

❖ maintain close links with key people in the wider community, whether they are workers in the statutory sector, service users, carers or from the voluntary sector;

❖ uphold ground rules in meetings and other communications, e.g. ensuring that clear and accessible language is used rather than jargon and that equalities issues are addressed;

❖ ensure that all parties participate in a constructive, frank and honest way, and work in the best interests of the UFM project;

❖ work to alleviate any mistrust or misunderstanding between service users and service providers.

Steering groups

In addition, steering groups may:

❖ take collective decisions and actively guide the project to the successful achievement of its goals;

❖ monitor the progress of the UFM project, receiving regular feedback from the UFM co-ordinator on how the project's milestones are being achieved, including ensuring the project is completed on time and within the agreed budget;

❖ assist the UFM co-ordinator and team if they encounter any difficulties in carrying out the project, using local knowledge and contacts and 'trouble-shooting' when necessary;

❖ provide expert assistance where necessary, for example concerning research techniques;

❖ maintain an equal balance between service users and staff through their decision-making function and through collective responsibility;

❖ work towards the sustainability of the UFM project.

Example of site visit questions and sample page of workbook

Sample questions on treatments and therapies

❖ Does the service provide enough information about the medication you take and its side effects?

❖ Does the service provide a range of talking therapies such as group therapy and individual counselling?

❖ Does the service provide a range of alternative and complementary therapies?

Sample page of workbook – question on medication

Rating 8: *Does the service provide enough information about the medication you take and its side effects?*
Interviewer's observations:
Service users' views:
Recommendations:
Does the service provide enough information about the medication you take and its side effects?

Rating:	1	2	3	4	5
	Not	Slightly	Moderately	Definitely	Extremely

Resources

Payment and benefits advice

Directgov website provides information on tax and benefits
www.direct.gov.uk

Child Poverty Action Group produces a handbook on benefits and tax credits.
Address: 94 White Lion Street, London N1 9PF
Tel: 020 7837 7979, www.cpag.org.uk/

Disability Alliance produces the *Disability Rights Handbook* and *Moving into work, A guide to the benefits and tax credits*.
Address: Universal House, 88–94 Wentworth Street, London E1 7SA
Tel: 020 7247 8776
www.disabilityalliance.org/

HM Revenue & Customs www.hmrc.gov.uk/

Jobcentre Plus www.jobcentreplus.gov.uk

General: user involvement, mental health, social care and public health

Directory of Social Change www.dsc.org.uk

INVOLVE www.invo.org.uk

Mind and MINDinfoline www.mind.org.uk

Mental Health Foundation (MHF) www.mentalhealth.org.uk

The Sainsbury Centre for Mental Health (SCMH) www.scmh.org.uk

Social Care Institute for Excellence (SCIE) www.scie.org.uk

Social research and service user research

INVOLVE www.invo.org.uk

National Centre for Social Research www.natcen.ac.uk

Service User Research Group England (SURGE) email: info@surge.scmh.org.uk

Survivor Research Network (SRN) (c/o Mental Health Foundation) see above

Service User Research Enterprise (SURE) c.ostrer@iop.kcl.ac.uk 020 7848 5104

Shaping our lives www.shapingourlives.org.uk

UFM Network www.ufmnetwork.org.uk

Useful reading

Directory of Social Change (2005) *Making People Welcome: The Sourcebook on Diversity*. 1st edition. London: Directory of Social Change.

Faulkner, A. (2004) *The ethics of survivor research – guidelines for the ethical conduct of research carried out by mental health service users and survivors*. York: Joseph Rowntree Foundation.

Fernando, S. (2003) *Cultural Diversity, Mental Health and Psychiatry: The Struggle against Racism*. Hove & New York: Brunner-Routledge.

Lowes, L. & Hulatt, I. (eds) (2005) *Involving service users in health and social care research*. London: Routledge.

Mental Health Foundation (1999) *The DIY Guide to Survivor Research: Everything you always wanted to know about survivor-led research but were afraid to ask*. London: Mental Health Foundation.

Rose, D. (2001) *Users' Voices: The perspectives of mental health service users on community and hospital care*. London: The Sainsbury Centre for Mental Health.

SCMH (2002) *Breaking the Circles of Fear: A review of the relationship between mental health services and African and Caribbean communities*. London: The Sainsbury Centre for Mental Health.

Lists of UFM project reports are available from www.ufmnetwork.org.uk or www.scmh.org.uk

General reading on research

Denscombe, M. (1998) *The Good Research Guide, for Small-Scale Social Research Projects*. Buckingham: Open University Press.

Blaxter, L., Hughes, C. & Tight, M. (1996) *How to Research*. Buckingham: Open University Press.

Hart, C. (1998) *Doing a Literature Review*. London: Sage.

General reading on statistics

Rowntree, D. (1991) *Statistics without Tears: An Introduction for Non Mathematicians*. London: Penguin.

Field, A. (2005) *Discovering Statistics Using SPSS*. 2nd edition. London: Sage.